W9-DGF-976

RESEARCH HIGHLIGHTS IN SOCIAL WORK 49

Co-Production and Personalisation in Social Care

Research Highlights in Social Work

This topical series examines areas of particular interest to those in social and community work and related fields. Each book draws together different aspects of the subject, highlighting relevant research and drawing out implications for policy and practice. The project is under the editorial direction of Professor Joyce Lishman, Head of the School of Applied Social Studies at the Robert Gordon University in Aberdeen.

RESEARCH HIGHLIGHTS IN SOCIAL WORK 49

Co-Production and Personalisation in Social Care

Changing Relationships in the Provision of Social Care

Edited by Susan Hunter and Pete Ritchie

Jessica Kingsley Publishers
London and Philadelphia

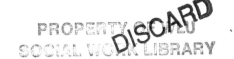

PROPERTY OF MLU
SOCIAL WORK LIBRARY
DISCARD

Research Highlights in Social Work 49
Editors: Hazel Kemshall and Gill McIvor
Secretary: Anne Forbes
Editorial Advisory Committee:

Prof. J. Lishman	Editorial Director – Head of School, School of Applied Social Studies, Robert Gordon University, Aberdeen
Prof. I. Broom	Robert Gordon University, Aberdeen
Mr S. Black	Edinburgh
Prof. B. Daniel	University of Dundee
Ms F. Hodgkiss	The Scottish Executive
Ms S. Hunter	University of Edinburgh
Prof. A. Kendrick	University of Strathclyde
Mr C. Mackenzie	Social Work Department, Aberdeenshire Council
Dr A. Robertson	University of Edinburgh
Ms K. Skinner	The Scottish Institute for Excellence in Social Work Education

**Robert Gordon University
School of Applied Social Studies
Faculty of Health and Social Care
Garthdee Road, Aberdeen AB10 7QG**

First published in the United Kingdom in 2007
by Jessica Kingsley Publishers
116 Pentonville Road
London N1 9JB, England
and
400 Market Street, Suite 400
Philadelphia, PA 19106, USA
www.jkp.com

Copyright © 2007 Robert Gordon University, Research Highlights Advisory Group, School of Applied Social Studies

All rights reserved. No part of this publication may be reproduced in any material form (including photocopying or storing it in any medium by electronic means and whether or not transiently or incidentally to some other use of this publication) without the written permission of the copyright owner except in accordance with the provisions of the Copyright, Designs and Patents Act 1988 or under the terms of a licence issued by the Copyright Licensing Agency Ltd, 90 Tottenham Court Road, London, England W1T 4LP. Applications for the copyright owner's written permission to reproduce any part of this publication should be addressed to the publisher.
Warning: The doing of an unauthorised act in relation to a copyright work may result in both a civil claim for damages and criminal prosecution.

Library of Congress Cataloging in Publication Data
A CIP catalog record for this book is available from the Library of Congress

British Library Cataloguing in Publication Data
A CIP catalogue record for this book is available from the British Library

ISBN 978 1 84310 558 9

Printed and Bound in Great Britain by
Athenaeum Press, Gateshead, Tyne and Wear

The editors would like to thank everyone who collaborated with Scottish Human Services (SHS) over the years, whether as users of services, professionals, planners or colleagues, whose wisdom and courage provided the inspiration for this book.

Contents

Figures, Boxes and Tables

CHAPTER 1

Introduction

With, Not To: Models of Co-Production in Social Welfare

Susan Hunter and Pete Ritchie

The purpose of this book is to explore the theory and practice of co-production in social work and related fields.

In this introductory chapter we define co-production as a particular form of partnership between people who use social care services and the people and agencies who provide them. Later chapters then provide examples of methods and services designed on co-production principles. The Endnote draws out some common themes and offers some suggestions about the future development of a co-production approach in the UK context.

Defining co-production

Co-production describes a particular approach to partnership between people who rely on services and the people and agencies providing those services.

Over the last two decades, partnership has become a constant theme in social policy, with a particular emphasis on formal and often long-term multi-agency partnerships. These partnerships address issues which are relevant to more than one agency or sector, for example urban regeneration, mental health, community safety or environmental sustainability.

Such partnerships are intended both to align the policies, priorities and efforts of different agencies with a contribution to make to the issue, and to encourage resource sharing. There has been a proliferation of partnership boards to promote social, economic and environmental objectives at local and national level – with a medium-size city such as Edinburgh typically having over a hundred partnership boards of different shapes and sizes.

Most partnership boards seek to include in their membership representatives from the relevant 'community' – whether a geographical community or a community of interest. Partnership boards operating in the social work field, such as a learning disability partnership board or a strategic planning and implementation group for older people, typically reserve a minority of places for representatives of service users and families. These representatives are sometimes nominated by broad-based, open membership organisations, and sometimes co-opted onto the board through more informal methods.

Both the partnership boards themselves and the arrangements within these boards for including the beneficiaries in the partnership process vary greatly in their effectiveness between 'collaborative advantage' and 'collaborative inertia' (Huxham 1996). At their best, such groups look beyond the distribution of service resources to locate their work within a broader social policy context, and service users participate as citizens and stakeholders with expert knowledge. At their worst, such groups simply pass the time while decisions on policy and resources are made elsewhere.

In recent years service users have also taken on a stronger role in the governance and operation of both regulatory and service-providing agencies. Many not-for-profit service providers include tenant or service user representatives on their board. Service users are recruited to work as inspectors for the Care Commission and the Mental Welfare Commission. Some agencies involve service users in staff training or in quality assurance. The depth and range of such involvement varies from mainly decorative to integral and effective.

While a minority of service users take up these partnership roles in policy-making and governance, all service users are affected as individuals by the quality of partnership in everyday social work and health care practice. For most of the people most of the time, being able to discuss, define and shape their own interactions with the services they use is central to their sense of autonomy, dignity and agency.

This book focuses on partnership at this individual level, for three reasons. First, much has already been written about the practice of partnership in strategy and governance. See, for example, Barr and Huxham (1996) on collaboration for community development; Harding and Oldman (1996) on involving service users and carers in local service; and the Joseph Rowntree Foundation (1994) on involving older people in community care planning.

While partnership in strategy and governance and partnership at an individual and family level are informed by the same values, they typically happen in different settings through different interactions and require complementary rather than identical skills and methods.

Second, the benefits of partnership at these other levels of the system do not always seem to trickle down to shape people's everyday experience of the service – we cannot assume that getting partnership processes in place at these other levels will ensure a culture of partnership in everyday practice with individuals and families. Conversely, there is something hollow about any system which promotes partnership in planning and governance without a healthy foundation of partnership in everyday practice.

Third, we are aware of several examples from different fields of social care where serious, grounded efforts have been made to design in partnership with individuals and families. We hope in this book both to bring these to wider attention and to draw out common underlying theories and methods – the 'family resemblances' between innovations in different settings and with different client groups.

In this book, we use the term 'co-production' to describe this particular form of partnership between people who use services and people who provide them. We distinguish this use of the term from its use by some authors – particularly in the US – to describe models where people undertake unpaid work in 'exchange' for welfare provision.

We choose the term 'co-production' as a conscious echo of the 'production of welfare' and 'social production of welfare' models developed in the 1980s by Bleddyn Davies, Martin Knapp, David Challis and colleagues at the Personal Social Services Research Unit, University of Kent. These models presented the service user as an object rather than subject of welfare production.

Making sense of co-production in everyday practice

After John's first day at the unit, the teacher said, 'Well, no problem with his reading.'

I said, 'How did you find out he could read when he can't talk?'

'Well, obviously, I got him to read a bit and then I asked him some questions and he pointed to the answers.'

'That's what I told the teachers in mainstream the whole of last year, but they wouldn't listen.'

'I've got a question for all of you – care staff, doctor, nurse, social worker, my friend here – when am I going to get my tin with my money back in my room?'

I said to her, 'What's that you're injecting me with?' She said it's just a pain-killer. I said, 'I've already had morphine and a general anaesthetic – do you mind asking me before you start injecting me?'

One patient here is at risk of falling and he can't break his fall so he has a member of staff with him at all times. Most staff can do it quite naturally – they walk beside him, or they link arms – but one member of staff walks just behind him and grabs him from behind if he looks like falling. I said, 'How would you like it having someone walking just behind you the whole time?', but he doesn't get it.

These examples illustrate some contexts for co-production in everyday practice.

The mainstream school could not reach a shared understanding with the parents of a boy with a label of autism about his ability to read and learn – so partnership in his education became impossible.

The man with a learning disability and a history of institutional living is making an appeal for partnership in managing his own money, while staff are concerned that he will keep spending all his money for the week or the month as soon as he gets it.

The woman in hospital after an operation wants to be treated as a person, not a body – and the man who is at risk of falling wants staff to be alongside him, not controlling him.

In all of these examples, there is an opportunity for improving welfare which can only be realised by services offering a different relationship with the person who needs help. Progress is made when services respect and seek to understand the person's world and see the person as part of the problem-solving team, not as a problem.

Co-production is an approach to service design and delivery which is informed by a distinctive world-view and which demands particular skills and methods to make it work. It is one way to tackle some of the deep-rooted malaise in the contemporary human service system.

What is the problem?

Many people are underserved by the human service system. Some of this results from the orientation and focus of services, with people's important needs not being addressed at all, or with services actually compounding people's problems – for example by increasing isolation, stigma and dependence. Some of it results from inadequate resources – either in the system as a whole, or in actually reaching the people who need them. Some of it results from poor methods or a lack of skill.

Unsurprisingly, the people most failed are those with least status and power, those who are least valued by society and have the poorest social networks, and those whose needs call for imaginative, flexible, coordinated, consistent and long-term responses.

Several different and useful approaches can be used to tackle this problem.

Philosophical reorientation

Some fields of social welfare have seen major changes of belief and direction. The social barriers model of disability and the independent living movement, the closure of large institutions for people with a learning disability, the shift from removing children from families to keeping children in families – these changes all involved a challenge to established thinking and policy. In other fields, such as prisons, the challenge to current thinking and policy has been unable to achieve a definitive shift from punishment to habilitation.

Such philosophical reorientations can also co-exist for long periods with services and systems set up under the previous regime.

Re-engineering delivery

This approach seeks to make the system more efficient at doing what it does. Measures include, for example, seeking to reduce transaction costs by merging or aligning agencies; setting targets to increase productivity; introducing new technology and procedures; contracting services out to private or not-for-profit agencies; and reducing demarcations so that each professional can do a wider range of tasks.

Higher standards, stronger monitoring

This approach makes expected standards of service explicit, increases transparency and holds service providers more accountable for performance. Independent monitoring agencies are less likely than in-house ones to reduce expectations to meet the available government budget.

Despite the well-known pitfalls (measuring what's easy to measure rather than what matters most, skewing activity towards performance indicators, encouraging a compliance mindset rather than internally driven quality improvement, focusing on minimum standards rather than excellence), this approach plays an essential part in service improvement.

Diversity and equality strategies

This approach recognises that the least well-served people tend to be those disadvantaged by age, ethnicity, gender, sexual orientation or disability. Specific measures are introduced both to raise awareness of this service bias and to change attitudes, procedures and service models to create more inclusive, equitable and responsive services.

Consumer empowerment

This approach borrows the language of the market and recognises that one of the causes of the mismatch between what people want and need and what they get is that service users do not have enough power to get what they want from the system.

Measures include ensuring better consumer information, so people have a better idea of what is available, not just what they have been offered; routing public funds directly to the service user so that she is seen and treated as a paying customer; appointing brokers to help people navigate the system; and encouraging independent advocacy to strengthen people's voice in the process.

The consumerist model is a useful way to challenge the traditional service delivery model, where professional and resource allocation power are aligned on one side, with professionals responsible for defining the problem as well as prescribing, authorising and implementing the solution.

The consumerist model emphasises that the professional or agency is providing a service to the person, not simply dealing with them as they see fit. It means that service users are entitled to receive a good enough service, that there is a formal or informal contract between the user and provider, that convenience, politeness, punctuality and acceptability are reasonable expectations, not just 'extras' at the discretion of the provider, and that service users can choose or change providers if alternative providers exist.

However, there are limits to the analogy between consumers in a typical commercial environment and service users in a typical service system. The analogy is compromised to a greater or lesser extent in different contexts by the relative powerlessness of many service users, by the fuzzy nature of the service, by people's reliance on public funds and by high specification and transaction costs.

All these approaches can and do make a valuable contribution to keeping services aligned with people's needs, and no one approach is sufficient. It is tempting for advocates of a particular reconfiguration of health and social work to promise that this will solve all the system's problems, or for advocates of direct payments to claim that once people have the money they will of course get what they need.

Similarly, co-production is not a magic fix. It does not dispense with the need for promoting equality, enforcing standards or improving delivery. However, it offers a different way to think about the relationship between the state, service providers and service users.

It differs both from the traditional public provision model, where the state is the administrator of a unitary system, the professionals are powerful experts and the service users are grateful recipients, and from the consumerist model where the state is the funder and market-maker, the provider agencies are competing suppliers and the service user is a free and informed shopper.

In the co-production model, the state has an important role in creating the conditions for productive partnership between professionals and 'problem-owners'. People who own the problem and professionals have a greater role overlap in defining the problem and developing solutions. This requires new thinking and behaviour on both sides, and whether this is described as a new 'script' (Leadbetter 2004) or a new 'dance' (Dowson 1991) it is a dynamic process with each actor or dancer influencing the other.

To take one simple example from the health service, illustrating the expectation that patients should simply present symptons and receive a diagnosis and treatment: it is still more acceptable for someone to visit their doctor with symptoms, without having thought about the possible cause and without having tried any form of self-help, than it is for someone to visit their doctor with their own ideas about the cause of their problem and having done some prior research on the internet.

A note on personalisation

Recent publications on the concept of personalisation (Leadbetter 2004) set out a distinction between 'shallow' personalisation – 'modest modification of mass-produced standardised services' – and 'deep' personalisation – with users becoming co-designers and co-producers of services.

There is considerable overlap between this concept of deep personalisation and our concept of co-production. Both recognise the limitations of the consumerist model. Both emphasise the centrality of dialogue or 'intimate conversation' in the process of co-production. Both terms are easily subverted. In our view, co-production has the merit of conveying a process involving two sets of actors.

Whichever terminology proves more useful, putting the concept into practice demands sharp thinking, imaginative model-building and honest recognition of the barriers to co-production in our current system.

Co-production is particularly relevant as an approach when the situation calls for long-term support; when it is important for this support to be highly individualised and 'site-specific'; when different people and agencies have to work together; when what is needed is likely to change over time; and when services are likely to have a major rather than minor influence on the person's quality of life. However, the attitudes and methods of co-production are more widely relevant to service design and delivery.

It is evident that co-production could (to borrow some of Maxwell's [1984] dimensions of quality) increase the effectiveness, acceptability and relevance of human services – and it is hardly a new idea. This suggests that there are considerable barriers to co-production becoming a core theme of mainstream philosophy and practice, since if it were easy we would all be doing it already.

We advocate co-production as an effective and pragmatic approach which can be defined in terms of some simple operating rules. However, these rules emerge from a distinctive world-view and we believe that a co-production approach is only likely to be sustained when this world-view is consciously adopted. Co-production should not be understood simply as a technical bolt-on to an existing service system. This is set out in Table 1.1 both to 'root' co-production and to illustrate some of the possible sources of discomfort with co-production as a philosophy rather than simply a model.

Table 1.1 Distingushing features of co-production

Operating rules	Underpinning world-view
People who rely on services involved in defining the problem as well as developing and implementing solutions	Recognising that different people interpret situations differently, hold different values and have different investments in a solution, and seeing the goal as securing a shared commitment to action rather than enforcing a single right answer
Tensions and differences between stakeholders discussed openly	Recognising that the interests of professionals and agencies are not identical with those of service users, and that saying one thing to people's faces while writing something else in a report is almost always in the interests of the professionals rather than of the person served
Focus on quality of life issues, not just clinical or service issues	Humility about the role of services in people's lives, and honest awareness of the quality and limitations of what is delivered
Engagement of people who know and like the person	Seeing people as part of a social network: and valuing the contribution of friends and family as much as that of professional staff
Use of ordinary language and settings as deliberate strategy to reduce power differences	Recognition of the games that people play to enhance distance and retain power
Engaging the wider community, and viewing this as a resource not a threat	Looking in from 'out there' as much as looking out from 'in here'
A focus on gifts and capacities rather than deficits	Actually believing that everyone has something to offer society

Skills and methods for co-production

A co-production world-view and approach demands, therefore, particular skills and qualities. Professionals are expected to work in a more open system with multiple 'frames' for discussion and action and multiple views of situations and goals. This calls for specific skills of facilitation, trust-building, reflecting, negotiation, resource-finding, interpretation and conflict management.

Professionals are 'marginal', to use Gerry Smale's term, operating at the boundary between the service world and the ordinary world (1998). This requires a high level of consciousness about role and accountability. Professional and personal ethics come under pressure when people make choices which carry high risks or which appear not to be in their best interest, and professional codes of practice will not offer a guide to action in every situation.

Above all, co-production exposes staff to ambiguity, uncertainty and challenge, sources of stress and discomfort which have to be balanced by strong and sophisticated support and supervision, whether from peers or agency managers. This outline of co-production is intended to serve as a theme on which the following chapters play many variations.

References

Barr, C. and Huxham, C. (1996) 'Involving the Community: Collaboration for Community Development.' In C. Huxham (ed.) *Creating Collaborative Advantage.* London: Sage.

Dowson, S. (1991) *Moving to the Dance – or – Service Culture and Community Care.* London: VIA.

Harding, T. and Oldman, H. (1996) *Involving Service Users and Carers in Local Services: Guidelines for Social Service Departments and Others.* London: National Institute for Social Work/Surrey Social Services Department.

Huxham, C. (1996) *Creating Collaborative Advantage.* London: Sage.

Joseph Rowntree Foundation (1994) *Involving Older People in Community Care Planning.* Research Findings 59. York: Joseph Rowntree Foundation.

Leadbetter, C. (2004) *Personalisation through Participation: A New Script for Public Services.* London: Demos.

Maxwell, R. (1984) 'Quality assessment in health perspectives in NHS management.' *British Medical Journal 288,* 1470–1472.

Smale, G. (1998) *Managing Change Through Innovation.* London: Stationery Office.

CHAPTER 2

It's about More than the Money

Local Area Coordination Supporting People with Disabilities

Eddie Bartnik and Ron Chalmers

The purpose of this chapter is to give a long-term evidence-based example of how the principles of partnership and co-production have become successfully embedded in the unique Local Area Coordination (LAC) support strategy initially developed in Western Australia and now implemented internationally.

The Disability Services Commission provides LAC support in the Perth metropolitan area and throughout all regional areas of Western Australia. The programme has been operating since 1988.

Local Area Coordinators (LACs) are based in local communities and each provide support to between 50–65 people with disabilities. This enables the support provided by LACs to be personalised, flexible and responsive. LACs aim to build and maintain effective working relationships with individuals and families in their local area.

Local Area Coordination is available to people with physical, sensory, neurological, cognitive and/or intellectual disability who are under the age of 60 at the time they apply for LAC support.

The LAC acts as a coordinator rather than a service provider and, as such, can help the person with a disability and their families/carers plan, select and receive needed supports and services.

LACs also contribute to building inclusive communities through partnership and collaboration with individuals and families, local organisations and the broader community. The overall aim of the LAC programme is to support people with disabilities to live within welcoming and supportive communties.

As the authors of this chapter, and as people who have worked in human services for 30 years, we continue to learn from our experiences and the ongoing research and evaluations that LAC is not only a very powerful way to develop and maintain an authentic and supportive relationship with people with disabilities and their families but also a means to gather evidence to help change the way in which communities in general, and formal service systems in particular, have responded to people with disabilities. Pete Ritchie at the Scottish Human Services Annual Conference in 1999 captured this idea well when he described LAC as 'a small-scale lever of large-scale change'.

Our aim is to present the LAC approach in a way that while recognising differing contexts for service delivery also emphasises the more fundamental or universal principles that underpin this way of working. We will refer often to the LAC framework, which is the vision and set of principles and strategies that underpins the approach. This framework relates closely to the notion of 'services as scripts' as outlined by Leadbetter (2004) in his writings on 'personalisation through participation'. The framework will also define many of the key elements of partnership and co-production outlined by Hunter and Ritchie in their introduction to this book, as well as the dynamic nature of a system where each party influences the other.

The LAC framework relates directly to the major policy frameworks in place internationally for disability services, for example in Western Australia (Disability Services Commission 2006), Scotland (Scottish Executive 2000) and England (Department of Health 2005). Some key common directions in all of these reports are the vision for a *good life* for people with disabilities, increased choice and control, more accessible and welcoming communities and the best value use of limited resources.

Some fundamentals underpinning reforms in Western Australia

The disability services system in Western Australia has had a major transformation over recent years, with the establishment in 1993 of a separate government agency called the Disability Services Commission. This department is responsible to the Minister for Disability Services and is guided by new legislation (Disability Services Act: Government of Western Australia 1993).

Disability now has its own separate focus in government and is not subsumed under a large human service portfolio such as health, welfare or aged care.

People with disabilities, families and community members are represented on the board of the Commission and have direct input into policy and strategic direction. Greater unity and shared vision in the sector gained through extensive strategic planning processes has led to increased political support and a succession of business plans of new government funding for disability services. Individualised funding and a state-wide network of more personal, local support through LAC are other unique features of the Western Australia system.

Consistent with the theme of this book, attention is focused on working at ground level with individuals, families and communities to make a practical difference. We have distilled a set of fundamental ideas that we believe underpin effective supports and services to individuals and families:

- Get to know people well over time and develop an effective relationship.

- Staff should be well connected to the local community and based locally.

- Hold positive values and assumptions about individuals, families and communities and shift focus and resources to strengths and prevention.

- See our job as building capacity, with key aims of self-determination and self-sufficiency rather than just providing a service to fix a problem.

- The need to ask the right question – 'What's a good life?' versus 'What services do people need?'

To summarise our views: we consider that the major reforms have been underpinned by two parallel sets of ideas, systems level ideas related to focus, community governance and unity in the sector, and a set of ideas about what constitutes a more effective way of designing and implementing supports at the levels of the individual, family and local community.

The history of Local Area Coordination in Western Australia

As with many successful innovations in social policy and social support systems, the LAC programme emerged from a combination of contextual, political and ideological realities. It was created partly out of dissatisfaction with existing services, partly from the drive and commitment of key champions, including families, and partly from the injection of new ideas such as the service brokerage experience in British Columbia.

The story of the origins of LAC and its subsequent development cannot be told without reference to the unique Western Australian context. With a landmass ten times the size of the UK but with a population of less than two million, the state poses significant challenges for those charged with the responsibility of developing sustainable support arrangements for particular sections of the community.

Local Area Coordination had its origins in regional areas of Western Australia in 1988. Over the next 13 years the programme was expanded until state-wide coverage was achieved and all people with severe and profound disabilities in Western Australia gained access to the service (see Table 2.1 below). The additional resources required for this expansion came partly from increases in government allocations and also from the redirection of resources from existing programmes. Strong leadership was required to facilitate the transfer of resources into LAC from these traditional programmes and strong will was needed to withstand the criticism that came from those affected by this change.

Prior to the introduction of LAC many people with intellectual disabilities were relocated to hostel or group home accommodation in the capital city or to one of the large coastal towns, a practice that mirrored the displacement of people with disabilities in other societies. One of the key objectives of the LAC programme has been to reduce the drift of people with disabilities away from their families and communities.

Despite the movement of many disability services to non-government organisations during the outsourcing drive of the mid-1990s, LAC has been retained within government. At key decision points it has been determined that LACs play a pivotal role in connecting individuals and families with the policy and programme systems of government and that this should not be lost in exchange for any benefits which may ensue from privatisation.

During its formative period LAC was viewed by many in the existing mainstream services as an oddity, a quaint and inconsequential feature on the service landscape. With the passage of time the programme has become an essential foundation for the sector and a major force for change and innovation in disability service organisations.

Table 2.1 Chronology of Local Area Coordination

Decision to trial LAC in one regional area of Western Australia (WA)	1988: LAC trialled in Albany
Following evaluation, decision made to phase implementation across rural areas (achieved in 1994–5)	1989–90: coordinator positions introduced in other regional centres
	1991: 40 per cent coverage of eligible people with disabilities achieved in regional WA
Decision made to pilot LAC in metropolitan areas in 1991	1991: coverage expanded to people living in Perth metropolitan area via a pilot project (ten positions funded by State Government, one funded by the Commonwealth)
Following pilot, in-principle decision made to phase implementation across all metropolitan and regional areas (target date June 2000)	1993: 27 coordinators located in regional areas and 11 located in Perth
Commonwealth Government decision to fund a pilot project to expand coverage to people with physical and/or sensory disabilities	1993: pilot conducted, involving a further 11 coordinators (full time and part time)
Following pilot, decision made to expand coverage to people with physical and sensory disabilities	1993–6: expansion of LAC in the Perth metropolitan area and growth of LAC positions in regional areas; by 1996 2478 people access the service
WA Government decision made in 1998 to fund a doubling of the existing service size, aiming to make LAC available to all people with disabilities across the State by 2000	2000: State-wide coverage achieved 2000–6: steady growth in the number of LACs to keep pace with the increase in demand for LAC services (approximately 250 extra people supported each year)
Major ministerial review of LAC conducted in 2003. State Government commitment to allocate funding to keep pace with future growth in demand for LAC services	2006: 135 LACs provide support to approximately 7500 people with disabilities

Sources: DSC annual reports and unpublished DSC information

The Local Area Coordination operating framework

Every system for providing assistance or support to people with disabilities can be analysed in terms of the philosophical or theoretical underpinnings that led to its design and implementation. The LAC framework is drawn from the simple proposition that the essence of a good life for a person with a disability is the same as the essence of a good life for a person who does not have a disability. This perspective leads us to ask the question: What makes a good life for any member of society? The answer to this question can reasonably be used as a sound starting point for approaching the task of building an appropriate system to support people with disabilities. It can also be used to examine the barriers that exist to reduce the potential for people with disabilities to lead good lives.

We have found that, when we ask the right question about a good life, the contribution and limitations of formal services and funding come more sharply into focus and the emphasis on family, friends and community increases. The framework has been developed to guide Local Area Coordinators in their everyday work with individuals, families and communities. While over the years changes and refinements have been made to the framework, the basic elements have endured. The framework comprises a vision statement, a charter, ten principles, statements about the LAC approach and a role statement for Local Area Coordinators.

Following an extensive process of consultation conducted in 2001 with individuals, families and key community representatives from across Western Australia, the LAC vision statement (a key component of the LAC framework) was revised to include a clear statement about the essence of a good life. The vision for LAC is that

> all people live in welcoming communities that provide friendship, mutual support and a 'fair go' for everyone, including people with disabilities, their families and carers. Developing a vision for a good life is a personal and individual matter. However, people with disabilities and their families throughout the state have expressed their view that a good life in the local community requires opportunities for valued relationships, security for the future, choices, contribution and challenge. (Disability Services Commission 2005b)

This faithful representation of individual and family views about a good life also assisted in bringing clarity to the role of Local Area Coordinators in the process of assisting people with disabilities to move towards this vision. This is reflected in the LAC Charter, another important component of the LAC framework.

The LAC Charter is to 'develop partnerships with individuals and families as they build and pursue their goals and dreams for a good life, and with local communities to strengthen their capacity to include people with disabilities as valued citizens'. Put simply, LACs stand alongside individuals and their families, initially to gain an understanding of their particular vision for a good life, and then to contribute to the realisation of this vision. This approach respects basic principles about the rights and natural authority of individuals and families to make decisions about their lives. The LAC framework enshrines fundamental principles about these rights. These principles (listed below) have been used to guide the development and operation of LAC.

- As citizens, people with disabilities have the same rights and responsibilities as all other people to participate in and contribute to the life of the community.

- People with disabilities and their families are in the best position to determine their own needs and goals, and to plan for the future.

- Families, friends and personal networks are the foundations of a rich and valued life in the community.

- People with disabilities and their families have natural authority and are best placed to be their most powerful and enduring leaders, decision makers and advocates.

- Access to timely and accurate information enables people to make appropriate decisions and to gain more control over their lives.

- Communities are enriched by the inclusion and participation of people with disabilities, and these communities are the most important way of providing friendship, support and a meaningful life to people with disabilities and their families and carers.

- The lives of people with disabilities and their families are enhanced when they can determine their preferred supports and services and control the required resources, to the extent that they desire.

- Services provided by government and community agencies complement and support the primary role of families, carers and communities in achieving a good life for people with disabilities.

- Partnerships between individuals, families and carers, communities, governments, service providers and the business sector are vital in meeting the needs of people with disabilities.

- People with disabilities have a life-long capacity for learning, development and contribution. (Disability Services Commission 2005b)

By building a commitment to these basic principles, Local Area Coordinators are encouraged and empowered to focus on natural, informal and community-based supports rather than moving quickly to engage formal services. The programme operates at the level of the individual, family and community. By focusing simultaneously on the goals, needs and potential within each of the three levels, the Local Area Coordinator can make a significant positive difference to the lives of people with disabilities and, at the same time, build more inclusive communities.

The role of the Local Area Coordinator

The preparation of a precise role statement for Local Area Coordinators has been a challenging task given the eclectic nature of the work performed by the LAC with its emphasis on responding to the individual circumstances of each person. The current role statement is as follows.

Local Area Coordinators:

- build and maintain effective working relationships with individuals, families and their communities

- provide accurate and timely information. Assist individuals, families and communities to access information through a variety of means

- provide individuals and families with support and practical assistance to clarify their goals, strengths and needs

- promote self advocacy. Provide advocacy support and access to independent advocacy when required

- contribute to building inclusive communities through partnership and collaboration with individuals and families, local organisations and the broader community

- assist individuals and families to utilise personal and local community networks to develop practical solutions to meet their goals and needs

- assist individuals and families to access the supports and services they need to pursue their identified goals and needs. (Disability Services Commission 2005b)

When this statement was revised in 2002 it was decided that it was not necessary to make a direct reference to the LAC role in the coordination of direct funding, despite this being an important and integral component of the

LAC programme. Direct funding has proved to be an effective support strategy within the LAC framework, and the ability to access relatively small amounts of funding has been highly valued by people with disabilities and their families. Consistent with the theory that underpins Local Area Coordination, however, direct funding is viewed as an adjunct to family and community-based supports rather than as the primary solution to meeting needs.

Examples that illustrate aspects of the Local Area Coordinator (LAC) role

- A man with a disability talks about one day living in his own home. The man, his parents and the LAC discuss a plan for some long-term strategies which assist him to identify and access the local networks which strengthen the opportunities for this to happen while maintaining his family connections.

- The LAC arranges for an experienced interpreter to explain guardianship issues to the elders of a remote Aboriginal community. This assists a family and the community to make decisions about a Guardianship application for a young man with a cognitive impairment.

- The LAC assists parents to plan for the transition of their young child into the school system. Through a series of home visits, and one important visit to the local school, the LAC assists with the preparation of an action plan to deal with all the issues associated with starting school.

- A man with a degenerative neurological condition believes that he is being discriminated against by the members of the body corporate at the block of residential units in which he is a tenant. He calls on his LAC for assistance to plan and prepare for his attendance at the next meeting of the body corporate during which he plans to express his concerns.

- The LAC assists a person with a physical disability who is having problems gaining required services from a local Home and Community Care agency. The LAC provides information about the particular agency, including services available and the eligibility criteria, and assists the person to explore how best to approach the agency. The LAC then attends the meetings and offers assistance where necessary.

- The LAC has used her knowledge of the local community to link the parent of a child with high support needs with another family in the local area. Through this connection arrangements are made for the child with the disability to be taken to school each day in the family vehicle rather than having to use specialised transport which has proven to be problematic.

- A mature woman with an intellectual disability who lives on her own has recently moved into the area and has become socially isolated. The LAC gets to know her and finds out she is interested in craft and attending church. Consequently, the LAC introduces her to a local church and craft group and she makes new friends who visit her and are able to provide her with support when needed. She also finds a valuable role in the church.

Local Area Coordination: Design and practice

Local Area Coordination can be described as a generalist or eclectic approach. It exhibits elements of individual coordination, personal advocacy, family support, community development and direct funding. The unique quality, and much of the advantage, of LAC derives from the mixing and blending of activities and approaches of each of these human service orientations as well as the intentional design of an ongoing personal relationship.

The aim of LAC is to make disability services and supports more personal, local and accountable, and to support local people with disabilities and their families in their local communities. The shape of the LAC support is deliberately kept fluid to respond flexibly to the changing needs of the individuals and families.

Local Area Coordinators are drawn from a wide range of backgrounds and professions (e.g. social work, psychology, education, therapy, nursing and community work). The key quality sought in a prospective Local Area Coordinator is a contemporary values base which reflects the vision and principles of the LAC programme. Wherever possible LACs are recruited from their local communities.

Each LAC works within a defined geographical area which may be a group of suburbs in a metropolitan area or a district in a regional setting. The role is to get to know and build a relationship with the 50 or 60 people with disabilities (and their families/carers) living within their allocated area.[1] Simultaneously

---

1   In 2006 the LAC programme was operating on a state-wide average ratio of 1 LAC to 62 people with disabilities.

the LAC builds knowledge and understanding of the local community as a basis for promoting inclusion and to expand the potential support base for people with disabilities. LACs work with children and adults of all ages and stay with people across the major transition points of life. It is the nature and quality of this ongoing relationship, and having one point of contact for local people, that is reflected consistently in satisfaction ratings with the LAC programme.

The level of assistance provided to individuals and families by LACs can vary significantly, from one family to the next as well as over time. The intensity of support is guided primarily by the wishes of the people accessing support from the programme and is negotiated on an ongoing basis. The critical starting point is in the establishment of a relationship between the LAC and the individual and their family. As part of the review process for the LAC framework, individuals and families across the state emphasised the following aspects of the 'LAC approach': positive values and attitudes; emphasis on relationships; effectiveness and a 'can do' approach; and personal–professional qualities (Disability Services Commission 2005b).

The relationship provides the LAC with an insight into the goals and dreams of the people they are supporting. If additional support is needed to help achieve these goals and dreams the focus will initially be in the area of local, natural, low-level assistance. More formal, structured services will only be considered if and when needed. Similarly funding to purchase services will only be considered when other no-cost options are unavailable.

Direct funding to individuals and families through the LAC programme varies from small amounts of non-recurrent discretionary funding administered directly by the LAC, through to small Flexible Family Support packages (up to AUS $5000) and then larger packages related to Intensive Family Support, Post School Options or Alternatives to Employment and Accommodation Support (all recurrent packages). The self-management of direct funding by individuals and families through LAC operates within the LAC framework plus an additional Accountability Framework (Disability Services Commission 2005c). The Commission's 2004/5 Annual Report states that 1431 people received these packages of support during the year, at an average cost of AUS $8248 per package. Successive audits and evaluations over many years have demonstrated the effectiveness and value for money of this graduated approach.

Local Area Coordinators also assist people to understand and navigate through the complex world of services and supports. Successive evaluations have found that this information and advocacy role is highly valued and can serve to reduce stress levels within families.

Local Area Coordinators approach care and protection issues from a strengths, self-determination and preventative perspective. This doesn't mean being naive about limitations and risks, rather it means starting with positive ideas and then introducing safeguards as required. They work closely with specialist services around vulnerabilities, reporting of critical incidents as required by legislation and any necessary safeguards.

In summary LAC has progressively replaced case management and social work/service coordination as the front line of the disability system in Western Australia. It is not just another layer and there has been a systematic process of readjustment and major reform.

The LAC 'script' (Leadbetter 2004) emphasises a more personal, local response with ongoing relationships and positive values around choice and control. Based 'outside the system' in local community shopfronts, and themselves having varied backgrounds, the LACs emphasise family, friends and community supports as the first step in achieving a good life. This new positive and preventative system is freely available to all eligible people living in a community and stands in stark contrast to the previous system, which was embedded in formal services and often rationed according to formal

---

Case study: Local Area Coordination in action

Late last year 19-year-old Isabel Wally travelled to Roebourne to meet her mother, Anne Wally, for the first time since her early childhood. Isabel, an Aboriginal woman, has multiple disabilities including cerebral palsy and intellectual and sensory disabilities.

After being taken into the joint care of the Department of Community Development and the Disability Services Commission at the age of five, Isabel was fostered for several years by a relative in Karratha who later moved to Perth.

At school Isabel befriended a local boy of a similar age, Cody, now 16, who also had disabilities. Cody's mother, Jo, noticed the bond forming between them and when Isabel's foster parent became terminally ill Jo became determined to honour her wish that after she died Isabel would not have to live in hostel accommodation.

When Isabel turned 18, Jo and her husband took over as her foster parents with a safeguarding plan which had been developed with the LAC. That plan included establishing and building a relationship with Isabel's birth family and Jo felt strongly that she should see it through.

With the help of Perth LAC and the Karratha LAC Jo began sending letters and photos to Isabel's birth mother Anne (who had been located by the LAC in Karratha). Eighteen months after taking charge of Isabel as her foster child, Jo realised that the Pilbara Beach Stay holiday home would provide an ideal holiday opportunity for Isabel to return to her place of birth (2000 km from Perth), with the chance of reconnection with her mother.

The Perth LAC arranged for Isabel to gain an experience of flight by organising time for her in the airline's flight simulator.

The holiday was a great success. On the second day of the holiday Anne came to visit. This extract from Jo's diary picks up the story:

> She is just like I imagined, but then I grew up here so have had the advantage of seeking many traditional Aboriginal women. What I wasn't prepared for was Anne's beauty, courage and strength. We talked, or as Anne says: 'yarned' into the night. I want to honour this woman, just for being here, after a 14 year gap.

> Anne shares her story. She tells me of the guilt and shame she has carried for years after relinquishing Isabel. I tell Ann, 'You are the bravest woman I know. You knew your lifestyle was unsafe and unhealthy for Isabel. It takes more courage to give up than to hang on.' She cries buckets.

> She comes back and has Neil (her partner) with her. He is kind. They both gave up alcohol four years ago and now support each other to live free from drink. Anne shows me the scars on her body from the years of abuse. What I am unhappy about are the inner ones.

> It took three days before Anne could hug Isabel. Thank you to the Local Area Coordinators for breaking through – for persisting and not giving up.

Isabel is now back in Perth with Jo, Jeff, Cody and their children. Anne is in regular contact by phone. Thanks to the sensitive and persistent efforts of the LACs and the remarkable strength of character of both her foster mother and her natural mother, the fabric of Isabel's family is knitting back together again.

Source: Disability Services Commission (WA) Update Magazine, 2002.

assessments and critical need. This LAC system correlates extremely highly to the elements of best practice recently identified by the Nucleus Group in Australia, as part of a national study commissioned by the National Disability Administrators (Nucleus Group 2002). Specialist services in Western Australia are highly valued but have been reformed and reintroduced in a way that complements and supports the more natural role of family, friends and community rather than replacing them.

Long-term evidence of the effectiveness of Local Area Coordination

Local Area Coordination has been underpinned by an ongoing series of evaluations at each key stage of development both in Western Australia and more recently interstate and overseas (e.g. Chenowyth and Stehlik 2002 and Lewis 1996; see Chadbourne 2003 for a complete review of these studies prior to 2002).

Two key themes have been consistent across all these studies. First, that LAC is highly valued by people with disabilities and their families and the general experience is of a high level of satisfaction and relevance. People value the personal relationship, positive approach and practical support to make things happen in their local community. The second theme is good value for money. The programme has low bureaucracy and per capita cost; small funding packages have been found to have a strong preventative effect; there is a strong alignment with strategic goals; and there has been a strong harnessing effect in bringing in a wider range of community resources.

In addition to the development of LAC within Western Australia, the programme was selected as a national case study of reform of government service delivery and featured in a publication by the Commonwealth/State Productivity Commission (Steering Committee of the Review of Commonwealth/State Services Provision 1998). The national profile started to grow from the late 1990s and the approach has now been progressively implemented in a number of Australian states and territories (e.g. Queensland, Northern Territory, New South Wales, Australian Capital Territory) as well as in Scotland, as part of the national Same as You implementation strategy, and in Northern Ireland. There has also been significant interest from areas of England, Holland, Canada and New Zealand.

During 2002/3 the Australian Labor Party in Western Australia, as part of their disability policy at the time of change of government, commissioned a ministerial review of the state-wide LAC programme. The rationale was that, after more than a decade since inception and now with full state-wide coverage, it was important to review the operations of the programme and to ensure that it was providing good value for money. The minister appointed an independent review steering committee to oversee the work of a team of consultants on the following four terms of reference:

- summary and description of the development and operations of the programme, including all previous research and evaluations/reviews

- feedback from all key stakeholders on the strengths and weaknesses of the programme

- value for money study

- synthesis of data and recommendations for the future.

Data was collected and analysed independently from approximately 900 people directly (670 individuals and families, 100 agencies, 26 key informants and 100 staff) and a further 1350 people indirectly, through previous studies. The overarching conclusions in the final report were as follows:

- First, on all measures of consumer outcomes, service coverage and cost effectiveness, the model has proven to be highly successful over an extended period of time. Successive surveys, reviews and evaluations have been independently confirmed to be methodologically sound.

- Second, increased demands on Local Area Coordination brought about by extensions to scope, role, coverage; a growing constituency; and increased demands for accountability, in combination, threaten its medium to longer term sustainability. (Government of Western Australia 2003, pp.64–5)

Of particular importance was the value-for-money study (Bartnik and Psaila-Savona 2003) which examined national benchmarks, the extent to which strategic objectives were met, preventative and multiplier effects, cost-effective operations and opportunity costs. Public data was used, which was then verified by the Department of Treasury and Finance. The independent conclusion drawn from this report and other data was that:

> Several external evaluations of both LAC in Western Australia and elsewhere – most particularly Queensland – as well as internal evaluations and the value for money study commissioned as part of this review, have confirmed that the LAC model provides value for money outcomes not matched by any other areas of disability services delivery. (p.70)

Following the review, a set of 40 recommendations for improvement have been implemented and the programme has been strongly endorsed for future budget growth funding so that new LACs can be appointed to population growth areas. Some important messages regarding limitations of the approach are as follows: the programme is only as good as the individual LAC that the person has, hence staff selection, quality and consistency is critical; if you give the LAC too many people to work with, you lose the personal touch and emphasis becomes too much on critical issues; too much bureaucracy and emphasis on funding takes the LAC away from core business and direct contact; and people from indigenous and culturally diverse backgrounds may require additional strategies in order to gain effective access.

Safeguarding and strategic development

The LAC programme in Western Australia has had a deliberate strategy to preserve core values and purpose yet at the same time stimulate and encourage progress and change. This methodological approach has been inspired by the work of Michael Kendrick on safeguards (see Kendrick 1997) and also the management text *Built to Last: Successful Habits of Visionary Companies* (Collins and Porras 1994).

We have found over the life of the LAC programme that there is a need approximately every five years to systematically review the LAC framework in order to keep it contemporary and responsive to the emerging strategic environment. We also believe that a framework needs to be a living document and a robust set of ideas that is continually challenged and refined as we move forward with a preparedness to change policies, procedures and structures. A strategic approach to risks and opportunities in the external environment is also necessary so that key supports and interfaces are maintained and the programme remains relevant and responsive.

The key focus in this chapter, however, is on the internal programme environment and the systematic approach taken to maintaining a high level of quality and human capacity. The major features of this approach are shown in Table 2.2.

Table 2.2 Local Area Coordination: Key elements of programme quality

State-wide LAC values framework	Realistic ratios enable a personal approach to be maintained
Careful selection of LACs	*Human-sized* units
Clear job description and high expectations of performance	Strong supervision structure and performance development system
Planned opportunities for regular interaction between LACs and their line managers	Systematic induction and training strategy
Open culture characterised by participation, feedback reviews and evaluations	Deliberate investment in leadership, new ideas and partnerships
Independent monitoring on national disability service standards	Strong care and protection framework and commitment to training

Quality and development, we have found, requires multiple investments on an ongoing basis and in the case of LAC a substantial investment in the values base and people involved. While emphasising a high degree of empowerment, personal approach and autonomy, we balance this with a strong expectation around accountability to the framework and agreed standards.

Reflection on Local Area Coordination as a major systems reform

There has been a radical change in the service delivery system in Western Australia over the past two decades. Local Area Coordination has been a driving force behind transforming a traditional service delivery system from one in which people were required to fit into the available services into a new system of building supports and services around people, one at a time, in their local communities.

The experience gained first hand by the Disability Services Commission in implementing the new LAC approach has also provided an evidence base that has been progressively translated into public policy. An analysis of the past three five-year strategic plans clearly shows a clear trend away from an emphasis primarily on service delivery and coordination (1995–2000) through to an increasing emphasis on strengthening individuals/families and carers, family leadership and welcoming communities (2000–5) and, most recently, citizenship and the importance of a sustainable community response (2005–10).

In public policy terms there is also a growing recognition of the fact that in Australia over 70 per cent of all care and support provided to people with disabilities comes from family and friends (Disability Services Commission 2005a). It is simply not possible for the government and formal service delivery system to replace this support and hence, from a business case perspective, it is essential that the informal system of family and friends is supported to the greatest extent possible. This necessity, combined with the strong value-for-money evidence for the LAC approach, constitutes a compelling business case.

In terms of implementation, there has been an ongoing tension involved in shifting appropriate resources and power from the formal service system back to individuals, families and communities. This has involved explicit recognition of matters such as natural authority and trust, as well as the changing role of professional and service staff to reflect this new way of thinking. We believe that an effective system has a good balance between formal and more informal strategies, where each are valued for their contribution and where individuals and families can choose the level of self-direction and responsibility that best suits them.

We have also found that fundamentally changing the system also requires clear focus and long-term strategy, rather than a quick fix. The primary importance of the vision for a *good life* and *welcoming communities* is at the forefront of this reform, along with careful design, implementation and evaluation to build the evidence for new ways of working. In the final result, however, what has mattered most has been the quality of support that has been delivered and that the strongest and most authentic advocates for the programme have always been the individuals and families that use it.

References

Bartnik, E. and Psaila-Savona, S. (2003) 'Value for Money.' Paper for the Local Area Coordination Review Steering Committee, Perth, WA: Disabilities Commission.

Chadbourne, R. (2003) 'A Review of Research on Local Area Coordination in Western Australia.' Consultant's report to the Local Area Coordination Steering Committee, Perth, WA: unpublished.

Chenowyth, L. and Stehlik, D. (2002) *Building the Capacity of Individuals, Families and Communities: Evaluation of the Local Area Coordination Pilot Program.* Brisbane, QLD: Disability Services Queensland.

Collins, J. and Porras, J. (1994) *Built to Last: Successful Habits of Visionary Companies.* London: Century.

Department of Health (2005) *Social Care Green Paper – Independence, Wellbeing and Choice: Our Vision for the Future of Social Care for Adults in England.* London: Department of Health.

Disability Services Commission (2005a) *Annual Report.* Perth, WA: Disability Services Commission.

Disability Services Commission (2005b) *Local Area Coordination – Family, Friends and Community.* Perth, WA: Disability Services Commission.

Disability Services Commission (2005c) *Local Area Coordination – Direct Funding Accountability Framework.* Perth, WA: Disability Services Commission.

Disability Services Commission (2006) *Strategic Plan 2006–2010.* Perth, WA: Disability Services Commission.

Government of Western Australia (1993) *Disability Services Act.* Perth, WA: Government of Western Australia.

Government of Western Australia (2003) *Review of the Local Area Coordination Program.* Perth, WA: Government of Western Australia.

Kendrick, M. (1997) 'Leadership and service quality.' *International Social Role Valorisation Journal 2,* 2 (Autumn), 62–68.

Leadbetter, C. (2004) *Personalisation through Participation: A New Script for Public Services.* London: Demos.

Lewis, G. (1996) *Local Area Coordination and Individualised Funding: An Evaluation of the Operation and Impact across Disability Types and Geographic Settings.* Perth, WA: Disability Services Commission.

Nucleus Group (2002) *Review of Current Responses to Meet Service Needs of People with a Disability and the Effectiveness of Strategies to Support Families.* Canberra, ACT: National Disability Administrators.

Scottish Executive (2000) *The Same as You: A Review of Services for People with Learning Disabilities.* Edinburgh: Scottish Executive.

Steering Committee of the Review of Commonwealth/State Service Provision (1998) *Implementing Reforms in Government Services – Case Study: Offering Direct Consumer Funding and Choice in WA Disability Services.* Canberra, ACT: Ausinfo.

CHAPTER 3

Co-Production through Encouragement

The Braveheart Project

James Mulholland (on behalf of Braveheart)

> *It has long been accepted that there is a direct correlation between deprivation and ill health. People in the most deprived sections of society are more likely to develop cardiovascular disease and, when they do, they are likely to die sooner than their less deprived counterparts.*
>
> (NHS Scotland 2004, p.12)

This chapter describes the Braveheart Project, a programme in Central Scotland to help older people with ischaemic heart disease to live better and longer. What was – and is – different about Braveheart is that it recruits and trains lay people, including older people and people with heart disease themselves, to work as mentors with people who have serious heart problems. The mentors are facilitators rather than teachers, recognising that people themselves have to make the changes in lifestyle and self-confidence needed to improve and maintain their health. Braveheart provides the information and encouragement to help people do this.

Braveheart is also distinctive in that it was designed initially as a demonstration project, with a randomised controlled trial to assess the effectiveness of lay mentoring. The results of the study showed that 'lay health mentoring is feasible, practical and inclusive, positively influencing diet, physical activity, and resource utilization in older subjects with ischemic heart disease without causing harm' (Coull *et al.* 2004, p.351).

Context

Scotland historically has had high levels of heart disease in comparison with other European countries. In the last ten years Scotland has seen a 30 per cent reduction in premature deaths and has started to narrow the gap, although rates have fallen in other countries as well. However, mortality rates remain nearly twice as high in the most deprived 20 per cent of the population as in the most affluent 20 per cent.

Lifestyle factors such as diet, smoking and physical exercise have a major influence – both individually and particularly in combination – on people's risk of heart disease. Levels of education, self-confidence and social support have a major influence on people's overall health and well-being, and on their ability to manage and improve their own health.

The Braveheart Project grounded its approach in the philosophy of Carl Rogers (1951). Rogers' theory of personal development emphasises the need to create conditions where people feel safe so that they can take on board new ways of seeing themselves and their situation. His thesis that 'the best vantage point for understanding behaviour is from the internal frame of reference of the individual' implies that people can only make changes in lifestyle and behaviour when it makes sense to them. He explains how we become defensive when under threat, and how this leads us to distort and deny our experience to hold on to our existing self-concepts. Braveheart put this philosophy into practice by using a mentoring approach rather than a teaching approach. If people felt safe, respected and supported then over time they would be able to change their sense of self and the way they lead their life.

History of the Braveheart Project

In 1996, after discussions between the Scottish Office, the Education Health Board for Scotland and Age Concern Scotland, it was agreed that an Ageing Well Demonstration Project involving ischaemic heart disease patients should be set up in Falkirk and District Royal Infirmary.

The project objective was 'to examine the effects and feasibility of educating and empowering older people with ischaemic heart disease to take responsibility for changing to a healthier lifestyle using trained senior health mentors. In this instance 'senior' denotes the fact that the health mentors themselves would be in the older age range, from 55 years of age upwards. Participants would be inpatients and outpatients aged 60 or over attending secondary care with a diagnosis of angina or acute myocardial infarction.

In addition to the current recognised standard level of care for heart patients some trial participants would be assigned randomly to mentoring groups, meeting every three weeks for two hours at a time over the course of a year. Each mentoring group would be made up of ten participants and each session would be led by two fully trained senior health mentors, one male and one female.

Initially it had been proposed that the sessions should be led by one mentor but in the dual interests of obviating the absence of mentors due to illness or other unforeseen circumstances and the need to cover any sensitive male or female issues it was decided that two mentors would be in the best interest of the project.

The trial commenced during 1996 with the initial recruitment of ten senior lay health mentors, a mixture of both men and women. These mentors undertook their mentor training during January/February 1997 and the first mentoring groups met in April 1997. The project began with 319 participants and 289 completed exit assessments. During the life span of the trial a further ten mentors were recruited and trained. The trial ended during the first quarter of the year 2002.

Control of the project

Overall control of the project was exercised by a management committee which included professionals from across the health spectrum and included representatives from Health Education Board for Scotland (HEBS), Falkirk Council, Merck Sharpe & Dohme (a major pharmaceutical company), Age Concern Scotland and the Project Coordinator. The committee was chaired by a consultant in geriatric medicine from within Falkirk Royal Infirmary.

The day-to-day control, organisation and running of the project, including the recruitment and training of mentors and ensuring an adequate supply of patient referrals to meet the statistical requirements of the project, were all the responsibility of the coordinator. This was an enormous task and to this end the coordinator's hours were 'protected' in that they were entirely funded for the project alone.

Patient referrals were as crucial to the project as the role of mentor. During the trial period patients were referred by hospital consultants, cardiac rehabilitation staff and family doctors. Initially some referred patients were reluctant to take part in the project, and to overcome this each and every one of them was personally interviewed by the coordinator and given a full and frank description of the project and its potential health benefits. This process was highly successful in resolving issues of doubt raised by the patients and in many cases created enthusiastic support for the idea of mentoring.

Core programme

The mentoring groups had a core programme which sought to bring participants and health professionals closer together by a two-way exchange of information in an open and non-threatening environment. Success depended on creating confidence in participants that professionals would listen to and support them in making decisions about improving their lifestyle, and creating confidence in professionals that participants would commit to implementing the agreed changes.

The core programme covered the following subjects:

- diagnosis – risk factors
- treatment for various heart conditions
- medication – which medication and why; importance of dosage
- healthy eating (participants were encouraged to keep eating diaries)
- exercise – walking, leisure activities, fitness classes; recognition of limitations and plans for change
- stress – recognition, avoidance techniques
- alcohol – recognition of 'safe' levels of consumption
- smoking – damage to health; cessation techniques
- cycle of change – regression not a reason for giving up but a spur to future success.

The core programme led to many associated subjects being raised by the participants which were personal to them and which because of the year-long commitment could be dealt with in some detail. The time span also helped to overcome the 'recidivist element' always present in the cycle of change.

Support to the groups was provided by visits from health professionals attached to Falkirk Royal Infirmary, such as cardiac rehabilitation nurses, dieticians, pharmacists and smoking cessation specialists, when requested by the health mentors. The professionals also set up a hotline for the health mentors which would provide answers to questions raised by participants at mentoring sessions, thus ensuring that response time was kept to an absolute minimum.

Whilst all this help was available to the mentoring groups there was constant reinforcement by the mentors of the principle of 'self-help' and the need for the participants to take responsibility, in partnership with medical advice, for their own lifestyle and its impact on their future health.

As the individual groups began to gel, the confidence of both the participants and the mentors grew, creating feelings of community and willingness by the participants to help and encourage each other. This community effect was further encouraged by the decision to ensure that as far as possible all the mentor meetings would take place outwith the hospital in venues (sports halls, education and adult learning centres, etc.) local to the participants. These resources were provided with the help of Falkirk Council.

Each mentoring group was encouraged to create a 'contract' which would govern the conduct of each meeting and which would be decided by consensus and was designed to be the first step, albeit a relatively small one, in the programme of the participants taking personal responsibility for changing their lifestyle.

These contracts would cover points such as:

- meetings to start and finish on time
- complete confidentiality about personal information gained at the meeting
- no smoking
- no bad language
- one person speaking at a time
- honesty and respect for each other's point of view
- acceptable venue.

The role of the mentor

At the outset of the trial, age (over 55) was seen as an important characteristic of potential mentors. They would have experienced and dealt with most of the same normal life challenges – marriage, children, setting up home, finance, education, health – as group members, and this would help to promote the ideas of self-help and partnership. This was a welcome change for some people applying to become mentors – instead of being seen as too old to contribute, they were seen as just old enough.

Most of those applying for training as mentors had themselves experienced varying levels of cardiac events, from angina to heart by-pass surgery, which also created empathy with the participants.

Mentor training was designed to ensure that mentors clearly understood that they were 'facilitators', not lecturers, and that they were not replacing health professionals but were working in partnership with them to create a group environment which would encourage and support the participants in following the advice of the professionals in leading a healthier lifestyle.

The dissemination of information, the right information, was seen to be of paramount importance in enhancing the health professional message and generating discussion which would lead to permanent positive lifestyle changes by the individual participants. Many participants regularly made the point that being armed with the right information also boosted their confidence when discussing their condition with their doctor or consultant and that they were surprised and delighted that in many instances both health professionals would actually discuss alternative treatment with them.

Continuous evaluation of and support to the mentors was essential and this was provided by the coordinator. Evaluation was based on regular one-to-one interviews with the coordinator covering all aspects of the group's progression through the core programme. Particular attention was focused on the group dynamics and any problems which had arisen with individual group members and how these had been resolved.

Support came via mentor meetings every six weeks, where all aspects of each group were discussed, problem-solving techniques analysed, information shared and a library of resources built up for communal use as required. These sessions created deep and long-lasting bonds within the mentor group, giving it a continued strength of purpose and commitment to the aims of the project.

Project evaluation

The evaluation of the original project was through a randomised controlled trial, with 319 heart patients selected to take part. Roughly half (165) were assigned to a mentoring group, while the other 154 were the control group, given standard health care. At the end of the year, 289 people completed exit assessments. People who had joined a mentoring group were walking more (over an hour more per week on average), were eating less fat and needed fewer outpatient appointments. Importantly, the project was successful in attracting and retaining participants from all socioeconomic groups, with a mean deprivation category score of 3.8 (where 1 is the most affluent 20 per cent of the population and 5 the most deprived).

From project to mainstream

Given these positive results, how could Braveheart continue to develop this partnership between people who use services and people who provide them?

During the Braveheart trial period a number of significant observations had been made:

- Patients responded better to diagnosis when they were treated as partners in the subsequent decisions being made about their health.

- Being given the right information to allow them to help make choices about the type and level of treatment they received or the changes they needed to make to their lifestyle was important to the participants.

These encouraging results led to the adoption of a new strategy to integrate the Braveheart programme into coronary heart disease primary and secondary care within the South LHCC (local health care co-operative) of NHS Forth Valley.

Unfortunately, before positive plans to pursue this objective could be put in place, the chairman of the project's management committee indicated that he would be standing down during the second quarter of 2002. At the same time the project coordinator also indicated that he too would be standing down as his contract was due to end in July 2002. The original funding stream would not be continued.

The chairmanship was offered to, and accepted by, one of the original group of lay people recruited in 1996, who had at this point six years of mentoring experience with Braveheart. A new coordinator took up her post during the first week of August 2002. Immediate and future funding issues now had to be dealt with. As neither the new chairman, apart from his mentoring experience, nor the new coordinator had any experience of working within the National Health Service, they very quickly had to form a working partnership which would allow them, with help and advice from the health professionals within the management committee, to create a successful bid for funding from the New Opportunities Fund by December 2002.

The evaluation of the resulting project, which ran from 2003 to 2006, again shows the positive impact of the programme in people's health and well-being. Out of the 90 people completing questionnaires, 40 per cent reported increased physical activity, 45 per cent said they had improved their diet and 75 per cent said they had gained confidence. Many spin-off projects have also resulted: cookery demonstrations to help people enjoy the oily fish which is good for their health, a Braveheart Plus group to help people meet socially once they have finished the formal programme, a walking programme and exercise classes at the local college. Braveheart has expanded into the neighbouring Clackmannanshire council area.

The project has attracted national and international attention and has made presentations at conferences in many parts of Scotland and the UK. However, despite its evident success, rolling Braveheart out into the wider health community was – and is – a very, very different proposition from its status as a scientific project.

As a small, pioneering project, Braveheart has created a great sense of commitment and teamwork from management committee, volunteer mentors and health professionals alike. This is always harder to retain as a project becomes part of the established way of doing things. However, the 'active ingredient' in Braveheart is its philosophy of respect and partnership – working with people, not doing things to them, starting where people are at and listening rather than telling.

The philosophy is designed into the programme: people meet for a whole year, giving time for them to make and sustain changes in their own way and at their own pace. They meet in a 'community' venue outside the health service, reducing the sense of fear and dependence which can be created in a hospital environment. While there is a core programme, most of the content of the sessions is created by participants, so they decide what is most important for them to talk and learn about.

This philosophy is encapsulated in the role of the mentor. However well designed the programme or the leaflets, it is the mentor's engagement with the group as a human being which is fundamental to success. If the group becomes a safe, supportive space then people will be able to face their fears. People struggle to change their diets and their lifestyle: mentors help them to get back on the horse when they have fallen off. The very fact that mentors are volunteers underlines the personal regard they have for group members. Mentors live in local communities, share the life experiences of group members and are grounded in the real world. One mentor brought in mince pies to celebrate Christmas – on the day the dietician came to talk about healthy eating! – not part of the programme, but certainly a part of the relationship.

Reducing heart disease in Scotland is a priority for the government and the health service, and has been tackled through investment in treatment and health education as well as anti-smoking legislation and a range of policy initiatives. Braveheart's contribution to this challenge has been to show that a person-centred approach, using local volunteers, can bring about lasting improvements in people's health and well-being following major heart disease. But, as one mentor commented, 'It's like any voluntary thing – your heart must be in it.'

References

Coull, A., Taylor, V., Elton, R., Murdoch, P. and Hargreaves, A. (2004) 'A randomised controlled trial of senior lay health mentoring in older people with ischemic heart disease: the Braveheart Project.' *Age and Ageing 33*, 348–354.

NHS Scotland (2004) *Coronary Heart Disease and Stroke in Scotland Strategy Update 2004.* Edinburgh: Scottish Executive.

Rogers, C. (1951) *Client-Centred Therapy – Its Current Practice, Implications and Theory.* London: Constable.

CHAPTER 4

Co-Production in Supported Housing

KeyRing Living Support Networks and Neighbourhood Networks

Carl Poll

Introduction

KeyRing supports people with learning disabilities to live in their own ordinary homes in ordinary neighbourhoods. Support is constructed from the input of a local volunteer, mutual support amongst Network Members, and community connections.

Perhaps the most surprising thing about this arrangement is that the KeyRing Community Living Worker offers a total of about 10 hours support a week to the 9 Network Members. This level of support is very small compared to staff input in traditional residential establishments. Carl Poll, who started KeyRing in 1990, here argues that the co-production elements of KeyRing Networks are the key ingredients of its continuing success.

Sixteen years on, it is hard to recapture the surprise and incredulity with which many greeted KeyRing Living Support Networks when the organisation began its work. KeyRing proposed that people with learning disabilities did not need residential care.

In the early 1990s the housing and support options available to people with learning disabilities were limited. Typically, people lived in homes with five or seven (and sometimes 20 or more) other people with learning disabilities. Residents generally had little choice about where they lived, who with, or who they were supported by.

Box 4.1 KeyRing leaflet for prospective members

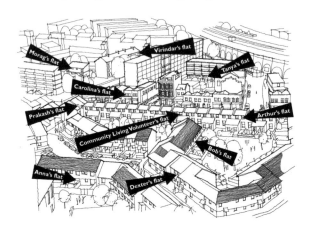

At KeyRing you can get help when you need it:

- KeyRing's Community Living Volunteer lives around the corner.

- They are there to help you.

- They won't boss you around.

- They are interested in what you think.

- They can help you to do lots of things – like reminding you to pay bills, or sorting out a problem with the DSS, or helping you to organise a party.

You are not stuck out on your own:

- The other network members in KeyRing will help you out.

- They live in their own homes around the corner.

- Everyone is in it together – everyone is a good neighbour to everyone else.

- There is a meeting with everyone once a month. You don't have to be friends with everyone. But you can if you want.

- If you are in KeyRing, you can have fun – like going to the cinema, going for a pizza, going to the pub, dancing, or organising a trip to France.

- And if you're ever feeling fed up, there's someone to talk to.

KeyRing's unique system of support is designed to make use of Network Members' own abilities. Ten ordinary properties are scattered around a small neighbourhood. You can walk easily from one property to another. Nine flats or houses belong to vulnerable or excluded people.

They have assured tenancies or their own property like anyone else. The tenth property is occupied by KeyRing's Community Living Volunteer (CLV) who supports Members on a regular basis. This arrangement allows KeyRing to build layers of support around the Network Members.

KeyRing leaflet for prospective members

Source: www.keyring.org. Reproduced with kind permission from KeyRing

KeyRing appeared on this scene and offered local authorities the opportunity to use an untested model based on the availability of about ten hours flexible, local support spread among nine disabled people, along with some back-up from a central office.

Approached from the prevailing social services viewpoint – that disabled people have problems which can only be remedied by the interventions of skilled professionals – it becomes easier to view these hours as a meaningless amount of one-to-one support. 'So someone with a learning disability who has had 24-hour support in the group home now gets an hour a week?' was the response of one surprised social worker.

There were many ways in which the work of the KeyRing Community Living Volunteer would stretch a long way. They live 'round the corner', bump into the Network Members on the street, can do meaningful five-minute pieces of work when they really count, are able to spot crises in the making, benefit from the information grapevine that operates within the Network and are available 'out of hours'. These are just some of the advantages. But even taking these advantages into account, other ingredients would be needed if the formula were to work.

These ingredients were the components of a co-production approach: understanding what people want; putting self-reliance at the heart of people's support; enabling mutual support amongst Network Members; and supporting people to make connections within the local community.

This chapter will argue that these co-production elements have been critical success factors in the development of KeyRing and Neighbourhood Networks (KeyRing's independent Scottish counterpart).

Preconditions of a co-production approach

Much has changed since the first Member moved into her own flat. KeyRing now supports 100 networks with about 900 Network Members. Neighbourhood Networks began work in 2002 and has 11 networks with 99 Network Members. Combined, the organisations have turnovers of about £3m. In 1990 KeyRing began with one worker – the author of this chapter – and a small management committee. The same worker negotiated with funders and local authorities and helped people carry fridges up their stairs.

At the conception stage in KeyRing, there was much guesswork about what would happen, and certainly some naivety and luck. Deepening understanding of the co-production elements in the Networks has taken time. While the picture of KeyRing's support came into focus, the slowly growing staff team learned to live with a great deal of ambiguity. They simply didn't know what would happen. Would detractors be proved right? It was common for professionals to issue warnings such as: 'He'll never cope. I give him a week. He'll be back' (e.g. to the group home).

Belief, commitment and determination were critical qualities in those early days. Arguably, these are qualities required in any radical innovation but they are not highly prized by statutory authorities, which generally seek assurance in advance that the system will work. 'What if something happens?' was a frequently asked question. KeyRing took comfort from knowing that for some people it was meeting – living in squalid situations and unknown to services, or responding with 'challenging behaviour' to institutions they found intolerable – things could only get better.

Another requirement for successful co-production was staff's attitude to the Members. New staff coming to KeyRing have often commented on the 'naturalness' with which people are treated. This came largely from gut instinct on the part of the first workers, rather than from a particular philosophy. People were treated with respect but not with reverence or indulgence. If people were to become more independent, clear reminders of Members' responsibilities were often needed. For those coming from more supported settings, this could be a shock. I remember an early conversation with a Network Member, who phoned saying: 'I want you to wait in for the electricity on Tuesday.'

'Why, what are you doing?'

'I'm out shopping with my friends.'

'Sorry, your look out – it's electricity or shopping.'

Over time, KeyRing has become more articulate in describing its value base. Key values and characteristics for KeyRing's approach are:

- listener – not presuming to know best about how to support people

- enabler – facilitating personal growth of Members and staff

- transferring resources and power to Members

- innovator – willing to swim against the stream to discover new means of support

- learning from experience and practice – willing to make mistakes in the interest of continuous improvement

- social entrepreneur – proactive in seeking to influence social care policy

- collaborator – committed to productive partnerships with other organisations

- strengthening communities – believing that support available within communities is at least as important as KeyRing's support, and that communities are the poorer without the contributions of disabled people

- equalities – staff behaviour must be: facilitating not dominating; learning not lecturing; progressively surrendering control to Members

- helping people to advocate – a greater role in society will be claimed by people themselves, not workers. KeyRing seeks ways of supporting people to claim that role.

Designing in co-production

Listening to what people want

The first component of co-production was KeyRing's willingness to listen to what people want. (It was only later that KeyRing termed this a social marketing approach (see Bruce 1998) and began to refer to people as 'experts on their own lives'.)

The chair of the management committee knew a group of disabled people in Wandsworth. In talking to these people about what they wanted in their lives, one thing emerged above all else. They wanted their own ordinary place to live and they were clear that they didn't 'want help all the time – just when we want it'. The idea that people would want help just some of the time led to a question about what they would be doing when they weren't using help. While some of the people in Wandsworth could be assertive and streetwise, they also had areas of vulnerability that could lead to serious scrapes. For example, Vic, one of the first Members, had arranged to wait for a friend on the street. He hadn't fixed a time, so waited for hours. The police asked him what he was doing, his name, address and so on. When he got confused and couldn't answer, they took him to the police station and treated him roughly. If this was what people could expect of the local police, how would they fare with unscrupulous people who might target them?

Self-reliance

How could KeyRing create a support system around such vulnerable people? The solution lay in choosing to focus on the strengths of the individuals, rather than to build a system to compensate for their failings.

Limiting the number of hours available from the Community Living Volunteer was essential if the system was to work. After all, who would not prefer to have a worker wait in for the electricity while we go out shopping with friends?

It takes time for those coming from more supported settings to appreciate the benefits of a deal around rights (your own home with secure tenure, ability to come and go as you please and do what you want) and responsibilities (having to pay the rent and comply with the tenancy conditions; treat neighbours with respect, and so on).

If Members did not have to fill a vacuum left by, say, former keyworkers in the group home, with personal responsibility and their own actions, many would clearly default to having staff do things for them. Ken Simons, in his evaluation of KeyRing (1998a, p.27), noted a range of Member responses reflecting this journey from dependence to self-reliance:

> It's her job [the Community Living Volunteer]. She's meant to do it.

> They try to give you experience, get you to do it for yourself.

> I do it myself. I only ask when I can't.

The Community Living Volunteer's role is an unusual one – part good neighbour, part facilitator, part advocate, part support worker. Discovering how to recruit good Community Living Volunteers has, like everything at

KeyRing, taken time to refine. An emphasis on understanding the needs of people with learning disabilities gave way to a stress on local knowledge or the ability to quickly establish community connections. Something that has remained a requirement is the ability to work in a way which does not steal the initiative from Network Members – negotiation not imposition. This is not easy: 'It is hard. I have to constantly tell myself it is their lives. I might not approve, and I will tell them what I think the consequences will be, but it is up to them' (Simon 1998a, p.25).

Building in self-reliance as a core component of support was, at first, a matter of faith and belief. But there was soon real evidence of people finding their own solutions. Problems were often reported to the Community Living Volunteer only after they were solved. Sometimes people used tactics which many of us wouldn't consider – like asking the fire brigade to help them get in when they were locked out (without getting charged). This and hundreds of other anecdotes suggested the creation of a virtuous circle of self-reliance (see Figures 4.1 and 4.2).

Members coined their own slogan – 'We can do it!' – and soon KeyRing began to talk confidently about mobilising the capacities of individuals as a key component of its support. It was only in 1997 that meetings with John McKnight, Co-Director of the Asset-Based Community Development Institute at Northwestern University, Chicago, and author of *Building Communities from the Inside Out*, provided KeyRing's approach with a theoretical underpinning, that of a gifts perspective as part of an asset-based community development approach.

As time went by KeyRing had an increasing expectation that not only would Members be able to manage their own homes and get around town, but that they might reveal singular gifts and talents. Singing, painting, relighting boilers, programming mobile phones and video recorders, writing, organising, transport, politics, geography, assertiveness, organising meetings, photography and cooking are just a few. All of these can be shared within networks. These skills and talents are now captured in 'gifts maps' – a simple tool to identify positive attributes.

One particular gift that KeyRing has come to rely on is people's willing-ness to speak in public – often approaching their subject with a directness that is more appealing than a professional presentation. Members are always part of the team which pitches KeyRing to local authorities and they are the people remembered as having convinced the authority to purchase. In this way

Members play at least an equal role in enabling other disabled people to get their own places to live.

By liberating the feelings of confidence and pride associated with being a competent and gifted person we can prepare someone to take place in the mutual exchange of wider community involvement. At KeyRing this begins with mutual support within Networks.

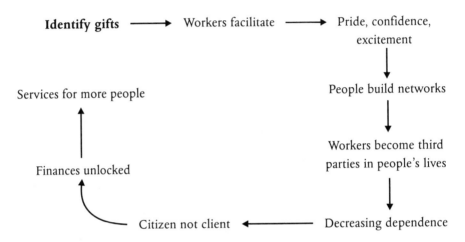

Figure 4.1 The consequences of working with assets
Source: Carl Poll, speech at Making the Community Connection, 2000.

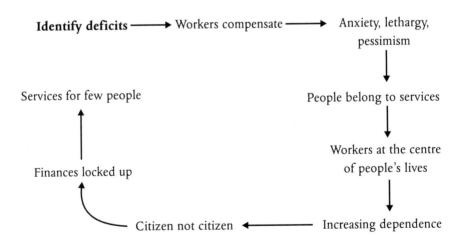

Figure 4.2 The consequences of working with deficits
Source: Carl Poll, speech at Making the Community Connection, 2000.

Mutual support

Another important factor in KeyRing's co-production approach was its comfort with the idea that disabled people may gain benefit from being together when they choose. In the early 1990s some regarded this idea as reactionary. More than one social work professional objected that KeyRing was forcing people with learning disabilities together. This, they said, was not consistent with the normalisation theories that held sway at that time: people shouldn't support each other because it's stigmatising for people to be in relationships with other people with learning difficulties.

Though politically correct interpretations of normalisation theories are less evident today, mutuality and association remain peripheral to most services for people with learning disabilities and are a missed resource. Even in 1995 the Department of Health's study of quality of life in various residential settings (Emerson *et al.* 1995) revealed that the quality of life experienced by people with learning disabilities rose in proportion to their number of contacts with others with learning disabilities. This was a finding which the authors, Eric Emerson *et al.*, considered to be one of the great surprises of the study.

Back in 1989 the relaxed and confident behaviour displayed by those people with learning disabilities who chose to meet up in the free-wheeling atmosphere of clubs offered by Generate (then called Wandsworth Rathbone) showed KeyRing that this association between disabled people offered another means of support which could be added to the design of KeyRing Networks – that of mutual support.

At first we were surprised (and pleased) when we saw examples of mutual support that had not been suggested by workers. One member showed off his pay-as-you-go gas meter. When we asked how he got it he said: 'Debbie's got one, and she went to the gas showroom with me.' This mutual support quickly became a part of the support mix that could be relied on.

Members of the Networks were always one step ahead in understanding this mutuality. From early on they referred to being in the Network as akin to club membership. This involved strong loyalty: 'I can't stand some of the people in our Network. But when we go out together, we're Hackney KeyRing!' said one member at the 1995 KeyRing AGM/party.

KeyRing staff resisted demands for KeyRing T-shirts because we wanted people to be ordinary. The idea of a T-shirt with the name of someone's support service just wouldn't do. We hadn't yet grasped the idea that Members were in an association – a group of people gathered voluntarily around a common interest. For members KeyRing was an independent living club where other people would know what it felt like to have your own place and from whom Members could draw strength.

An independent evaluation by Paradigm in 2002 (Kinsella 2002) confirmed this observation:

> There is a very strong feel amongst tenants[1] that they 'own' KeyRing. In business speak, there is a very strong brand loyalty. Many tenants are fiercely proud of their association with KeyRing. We found that many tenants see it as a badge of honour, enhancing their own status and self-esteem. Whilst often such things seem small and insignificant, items such as KeyRing keyrings, calendars etc. are prized and valued... Our feeling was that some tenants see it more as a club or association rather than a service. We doubt whether any other service could lay such a claim as that. (p.9)

Though Members were more sophisticated in their understanding of their membership than staff, KeyRing had provided the structural arrangement for this 'club'. From the outset KeyRing insisted that Members meet together at least once a month. The substance of these meetings was up to local Members, and it is perhaps this loose brief which enabled Members to discover and shape this associational function of KeyRing membership.

Some meetings are social – organising meals and trips abroad – others can be focused on shared problems, such as safety in the area. Some are more lively and active than others. Like any group, meetings must serve a purpose if they are to survive. The success of some network meetings is attributed by Kinsella to:

> a mixture of an enticing enough venue, the willingness and commitment of tenants, and the ability of the Community Living Volunteer to engage with, motivate and support tenants to attend. In particular, network meetings seemed to be most popular when there was a significant social element to them (2002, p.10)

It appears that the community-building motto 'don't have a meeting if you can have a party' is true in this case.

---

1   This evaluation refers to KeyRing 'tenants'. KeyRing owns no housing and Network Members are not tenants in the formal sense. Nonetheless, people were called tenants until they voted to be called Network Members shortly after the evaluation.

Another way of building in mutual support is through a Member contract, in which the willingness to help another Member if they need it is a requirement of membership. This requirement is illustrated by suggesting that, if one Member knows another is ill, the first should call by to see if the other Member needs any shopping or other help. This idea is readily understood and accepted. In practice people help each other a great deal. From trading (one Member tidies another's garden while that person prepares a meal) to gifts (furniture makes its way round a network, one person passing it to the next as they buy new), to moral support (a group gathering each evening to support someone whose flat was burgled). It is impossible to calculate the value this adds to the support people have received. There are certainly tens of thousands of examples of such practical and emotional help.

Community connections

In parallel to adopting an asset-based approach to individuals, KeyRing made a choice to take a positive view of the neighbourhoods in which Networks were sited. It was expected that Members would have ordinary relations with their neighbours and would make full use of community resources.

Locations of most of the Networks are on ordinary – some may say tough – estates. This raised some objections from social work professionals who considered that 'valued' neighbourhoods were only to be found in high-cost, leafy suburbs.

KeyRing's own judgement was that, while Members faced all kinds of challenges in living in ordinary places, they were, for the most part, able to learn from difficulties, maintain their place in the community and develop their abilities. In 1998, though, Ken Simons reported that:

> Around three-quarters of the tenants interviewed talked in positive terms about the local neighbourhood. In some situations tenants had developed significant relationships with people outside the network.

> However, nearly half the tenants also reported having problems with local people, including tensions with neighbours, harassment by relative strangers, and some deliberate targeting of vulnerable tenants. (pp.3–4)

He goes on to add that KeyRing had responded by:

- developing an audit for use in neighbourhoods where a new network is being considered

- helping individuals to develop defensive strategies
- liaising with local housing services, if necessary getting people re-housed in the locality
- support for tenants to take action against perpetrators
- ensuring access to services like victim support. (Simons 1998b)

In addition to defensive strategies and support to victims, KeyRing then adopted a more consistent approach to mapping positive features in the community: good people, associations and groups, 'third places' (good places to meet like friendly pubs), organisations and other resources.

A planned approach to mapping communities was one of the benefits of working with John McKnight. His emphasis on community capacity inventories (see, for example, McKnight and Kretzmann 1999) led to KeyRing-wide mapping efforts and an ever greater focus on the potential of Network Members to make important contributions to the local community. Neighbourhood Networks Members recently took this mapping a stage further by organising a local history project, interviewing local people and recording their memories of life around Bellshill in North Lanarkshire.

While mapping of local assets has become a standard activity in KeyRing, good local knowledge had always been a benefit of having a Community Living Volunteer who shared the experience of living in a particular neighbourhood. A Community Living Volunteer told this story:

> Jack had got friendly with a younger group on the estate – they were Somali and they were into kick-boxing. Jack got out of his depth and one night very late they were kick-boxing his front door. He was scared and phoned me. I went and asked them what they thought they were doing.

When asked if she was afraid to do this at nearly midnight, she replied: 'I just knew they wouldn't do anything to me as a woman. Anyway, they know that we all know the same people on the estate.' It is hard to imagine that a co-production approach in this context could be supported by visiting workers.

John McKnight, in a meeting with KeyRing, also suggested that a major outcome from this co-production approach was that KeyRing had created 'walking-around space' for people who were normally controlled by services. By 'walking-around space' he meant that KeyRing had found a way of working with people without imposing, such that they became confident enough to navigate the local community on their own, and that KeyRing had persuaded local authorities to have confidence in individuals' ability to do this without being hemmed in by risk assessments.

Sal and John illustrate 'walking-around space' with their story of how, on their wedding anniversary, they were surprised by a knock at their door and were whisked off in a limousine to a West-End hotel. There was a big meal with lots of people. Speeches were made, and they came home with a cheque. Who arranged it? John just says: 'It was Fred down the market' (where John gets in teas for stallholders).

Sal and John made these connections because of their own unique qualities. The virtue of co-production here is that Sal and John did something that service workers would have been unable to achieve. It wasn't just that workers would be hard pressed to orchestrate such an elaborate event but, more importantly, they could not have established Sal and John's relationships with ordinary local people.

'Walking around' for people with learning disabilities is often restricted because of the fear on the part of statutory services of *something happening*. English Government policy in this area now sets a challenge that statutory authorities must support initiatives enabling services to be less risk-averse (for example, Department of Health 2005; Prime Minister's Strategy Unit 2005). While local authorities struggle to turn around risk-averse service cultures, Members at KeyRing, in running their own workshop on risk at a conference, are pragmatic: 'There's trouble everywhere. If you look for it, you'll find it. We don't look for it.'

With the support of Community Living Volunteers, Network Members have often established good relationships with local police forces and are able to enlist their support on questions of safety. A Community Police Officer in Bristol supported Members who were concerned about young people using a derelict flat in their block to take drugs. Members organised a letter from residents in the block and sent it to the Council. A new security system was installed.

There is no explicit co-production contract with local people about the 'inclusion' of Members within community activities. This would contradict KeyRing's insistence that people with learning disabilities should have the right to ordinary housing as any other citizens. However, if KeyRing learned of a potentially supportive local group, we would discuss the setting up of the

Network as part of the neighbourhood audit. A residents' group in Bristol responded: 'We'll keep an eye out for those folk.'

But, unlike some current views of 'inclusion', which see communities solely in a supportive role to disabled people, KeyRing emphasises Members' ability to contribute to their neighbourhood. While this reciprocal relationship is not stated in the day-to-day dealings between Members and other people in the community, it is part of the implicit currency of community exchange. Michael Young and Gerard Lemos write that mutual aid is a basic building block of community:

> The first and most humble meaning [of mutual aid] is of more or less simultaneous reciprocity between two people. A looks after B when A is ill and B looks after A when A is ill.

> The second and less humble meaning is lagged reciprocity... Friends and neighbours might help one another...with no immediate return, but with strong implicit presumption of help to be returned at an unspecified moment of future need.

> The third...meaning is where mutuality is multilateral – three ways, or four ways, or n-ways. A helps B. B helps C. C helps A. This multilateral aid can be stretched to include millions of people who are unknown, but although unknown, contribute to the welfare of each and every one of us. (Young and Lemos 1997, p.9)

KeyRing has high expectations of Members. Increasingly it has emphasised an agenda around citizenship and participation in the wider community and many have responded. Their activities range from helping out neighbours to writing to the Council about safety in the area. Members on one estate have become key members of a consultation group on improvements on the estate. Elsewhere, Julie met a woman walking her dog. Julie is shy and distrusts people, but got to know the woman and moved in with her for a short time after being in hospital. Julie looks after the woman's dog when she is away.

A good number of KeyRing Members take part in Timebanks and, in one location, are leading members. Timebanks are local time exchanges in which timebankers can bank an hour for, say, keeping someone company, and withdraw an hour of DIY help from someone else.[2] One Member became chair of the tenants' association. Some members, harassed by local youth, made a mature response. They lobbied the Council to reopen a youth club – 'There's nothing for the young people round here,' they wrote.

There are thousands of examples of such wider community mutual aid in which Members are important contributors and beneficiaries: 'the payoff comes from an analysis of people's lives. Compared to most people with learning difficulties being supported to live in the community, KeyRing tenants are community resource and relationship rich' (Kinsella 2002, p.15).

Advantages and limitations

While many of the advantages of KeyRing's model for co-production are set out above, it remains to pick out one overarching advantage – that of the relationship between cost and outcomes. First, though, a consideration of possible limitations.

The Living Support Network is a model. It is artificial and does not suit all people. Because of KeyRing's particular interest in those people with learning disabilities who hover at the edge of eligibility for social services, the model was designed around those with relatively good skills. This raises a question of its usefulness to other groups of people who need support to live independently.

Over time, though, KeyRing has discovered that there are many ways to overcome skills deficits, and that a better determinant of success is motivation – a quality available to people whatever the nature or extent of their disability. KeyRing maintains that, because of the flexibility of the Network arrangement, it could be useful to, say, older people, those with mental health problems, refugees and others.

Another suggestion is that this is an urban model. KeyRing has tried Networks in two rural locations – one in a small town and one dispersed around a wide area. While there are certainly different challenges in these areas – poor public transport, little social housing and dependence on a few local organisations for partnership working (which may not be sympathetic to KeyRing's aims) – these problems are not connected to the validity of a co-production approach. KeyRing suggests that benefits of co-production such as pride in

2   For more information on timebanks, see www.timebanks.co.uk.

making a contribution, a sense of belonging and increasing independence are universally desirable.

In the dispersed rural Network, KeyRing found it difficult to recruit Network Members. Though social services had made the judgement that there would be sufficient referrals, only two or three people joined the Network over a period of nearly three years. KeyRing has responded by widening the scope of membership to people with physical disabilities, people with mental health problems and people with sensory impairments. The Network is now running well with good levels of mutual support.

A further limitation – externally imposed – remains the perception of statutory authorities. The perception by some that this way of working is an extremely risky venture remains a significant obstacle, although KeyRing now works in over forty local authority areas and Neighbourhood Networks in four.

Perhaps more significant still is the poor fit of KeyRing's model with the regulatory framework. KeyRing has managed to keep outside the Standards for Residential Care and for Domiciliary Care (though Neighbourhood Networks needed to register as a Housing Support Service with the Scottish Care Commission). Both organisations, though, receive funding from Supporting People, and both struggle to demonstrate the benefits of their approach through Supporting People's Quality Assurance Framework. This performance framework, in essence, measures worker outputs rather than outcomes for Members. The style of working of Community Living Volunteers – working with the grain of people's wishes, rather than imposing solutions, and keeping in the background as much as possible – is out of step with a framework which measures how much time a worker spends enabling people to, for example, change a light bulb. This becomes problematic when evaluations of KeyRing produce statements such as 'I did that myself. No one helped me.' KeyRing celebrates such benefits of co-production. A Supporting People Monitoring Officer may take a different view.

This divergence of attitude comes from two world-views. KeyRing's is that individuals and communities are full of resources and capacities, and that the task of the sensible support agency is to help people mobilise these. The counter-view still dominates the funding streams for social care, the service world and, indeed, the world of community development: that disabled people and communities have deficiencies which only the services of skilled professionals can repair.

We know where we arrive if we adopt the second view. We arrive where we are now, with people who use social care disempowered and marginalised in the process of their own care plans and support arrangements. This means the loss of their contribution to their own and others' support, and to the community at large. It is also an expensive process and leads to services for the few.

In contrast the incorporation of co-production by KeyRing means that people become stronger and more independent. They need less support from staff. People feel better about themselves and their future. They become citizens and contributors to community. There is a cost implication here. The two organisations charge relatively little, KeyRing £3500, Neighbourhood Networks £4300 per annum, to support one Network Member. Residential care placements vary in cost. But a typical individual placement costs around £40,000. For this sum membership in KeyRing or Neighbourhood Networks would be available for about ten people. Put crudely: ten citizens for the cost of support to one service user.

The case for such co-production approaches to the support of disabled people becomes yet stronger when seen in the context of the Government's move towards personal budgets. A series of policy documents, including the White Paper *Our Health, Our Care, Our Say*, outline a new kind of social care system, one in which control over funding and the arrangement of support is passed from commissioners and support providers to disabled people and their supporters. A blueprint for a new social care system, Self-Directed Support, has already been developed and tested by in Control.[3] Speaking at the launch of a report on in Control's pilot work (Poll *et al.* 2006), Care Services Minister Ivan Lewis said that:

> It was always wrong that power and control was in the hands of providers and professionals instead of those who use support. Self-Directed Support is the direction of travel. It's about values and mission, about the kind of society we want to live in. It's about social justice.

The transfer of power and control over funding and support to disabled people has significant implications for providers of support. In a support market driven for the first time by disabled people, co-production may well become a prerequisite for those who are looking for customer-oriented providers. Those

---

3   For more information on in Control, see www.in-control.org.uk.

providers that continue to design services on a take-it-or-leave-it basis may find themselves without a role in the future system.

References

Bruce, I. (1998) *Charity Marketing – Meeting Need through Customer Focus.* London: ICSA.

Department of Health (2005) *Independence, Well-Being and Choice: Our Vision for the Future of Social Care for Adults in England.* London: Department of Health.

Emerson, E., Robertson, J., Gregory, N., Hatton, C. *et al.* (1995) *Quality and Costs of Community-Based Residential Supports, Village Communities, and Residential Campuses in the United Kingdom.* London: Department of Health.

Kinsella, P. (2002) *Report of Review of KeyRing.* Paradigm, unpublished.

McKnight, J. and Kretzmann, J.A. (1999) *Guide to Mapping and Mobilising the Associations in Local Neighborhoods.* Chicago, IL: ACTA Publications.

Poll, C., Duffy, S., Hatton, C., Sanderson, H., Routledge, M. (2006) *A Report on in Control's First Phase 2003–2005.* London: in Control.

Prime Minister's Strategy Unit (2005) *Improving the Life Chances of Disabled People.* London: Prime Minister's Strategy Unit.

Simons, K. (1998a) *Living Support Networks – An Evaluation of the Services Provided by KeyRing.* Brighton: Pavilion Publishing/Joseph Rowntree Foundation.

Simons, K. (1998b) 'Low Support' Options for People with Learning Difficulties: Findings. May. York: Joseph Rowntree Foundation.

Young, M. and Lemos, G. (1997) *The Communities We Have Lost and Can Regain.* London: Lemos and Crane.

CHAPTER 5

Co-Production

Support for Self-Employment

Jane Pagler

This chapter is about the work that I undertake as a client adviser for Enter at Disability Wales (Enter DW), supporting people with impairments to set up their own businesses. The chapter describes the origins of the project before providing some examples of the work undertaken and businesses supported with individual case studies.

Disability Wales is the national association of disability groups striving to achieve rights, equality and choice for all disabled people in Wales. Since its establishment in 2001 the Enter DW client support activities have been focused on empowering disabled people with information, advice, business idea development and the skills essential for business success. Enter DW believe any programme to promote self-employment amongst disabled people must address cultural, support and physical barriers which limit the participation of disabled people in business start-ups.

Enter DW services are managed and delivered by disabled people. The client advisers are all people with impairments who have established their own businesses, so the co-production is disabled people assisting other people with disabilities to explore their business ideas. The client advisers are a diverse and talented group, with backgrounds in, for example, banking, the law, the civil service and politics.

The impetus for the work undertaken by Enter DW is not from social care but from Potentia, a European-funded project managed previously by the Welsh Development Agency, now incorporated within the Department of Enterprise, Innovation and Networks at the Welsh Assembly Government, a project with the aim of supporting people from under-represented groups into self-employment. The key groups supported by the Potentia project are women and lone parents, 18–30-year-olds, over 50s, minority ethnic groups, disabled people and Welsh speakers.

Unlocking the enterprise potential of these six key groups is an integral part of the Entrepreneurship Action Plan for Wales with Potentia partners acting as a bridge between the client and mainstream business support providers. Research indicates that certain groups require greater support at the pre-business phase and Potentia acts as the catalyst for this early business development.

Enter DW is funded through the Potentia project and helps potential businesses started by people with impairments to navigate through the complexities of doing business in increasingly complex environments. They provide practical and informed guidance to harness and develop the talent pool of entrepreneurs with impairments.

Each of the Potentia partners has taken a different approach to providing support, with some agencies employing specific business advisers whilst others rely on a variety of self-employed business people and consultants with appropriate experience and skills. Enter DW decided to contract for a minimum of four days per month with self-employed people, all of whom have impairments, to provide pre-start-up business advice and support to potential entrepreneurs.

Although I had originally trained as a social worker 25 years ago, I had more recently completed an MBA in public service management and worked as chief executive of a large charity. I also had several years' experience of lecturing on a Taught Doctorate and Masters Degree in Management of Social Care. I had recently set up my own consultancy business when I saw the advert for the contract.

I was pleased to be successful in gaining a contract and have now been doing the work for over three years. The approach is positive and motivational, with the client specifying what they want to do and the pace at which they want to proceed. The difference to the traditional public service provision model is refreshing, this being recently demonstrated when I was asked by a social care worker at an activity centre if I was a potential entrepreneur's 'support worker'. The potential entrepreneur is determined to set up his own business and leave the activity centre and we agreed that in future we will meet in a more business-like environment.

The case studies are typical of the work that I undertake. Whilst the majority of people go on to self-employment, the process can also successfully identify the amount of work and commitment required, which assists people who had not accurately estimated this to make their decisions about whether to proceed. Similarly some people who investigate the options go on to employment, and this can be a positive outcome, as in case study 5. There are also examples of people who listen to the advice but decide not to follow it, and whose businesses subsequently experience difficulty, but these are fortunately in the minority.

Case study 1

C's interest in African drums started in Japan in 2000. On returning to Wales in 2003 he set his sights on becoming self-employed as a drum tutor and performer. C started doing voluntary work with youth clubs around his home town with the aim of introducing drumming onto the curriculum.

C sought the assistance of Enter DW for support in setting up his business. The assessment process identified the business idea, the supports needed and any potential barriers. As C had the basic drumming equipment with which to start, capital was not required, but financial support was important whilst C was establishing such an unusual business. His impairment restricts the carrying of his drums so solutions were investigated. C also had to take caring responsibilities into account.

C 'test traded' for six months on the New Deal for Musicians scheme, whereby he could retain his incapacity benefit whilst testing the viability of his business idea. The Enter DW Client Adviser also supported C on issues such as insurance advice and Access to Work applications for support with transporting the drums.

The main focus for his business idea is youth clubs, as C feels the clubs offer a limited range of activities. C said: 'I am bringing something new which involves young people developing skills such as teamwork and co-operation.' Future plans for the business include setting up a musical exchange programme between the youth clubs in his home area and Japan. In 2005 a team of drummers he trained won the local Youth Service Talent Show.

C is now successfully supporting himself with his own business, with the youth development and school work proving more lucrative than performing with his own band.

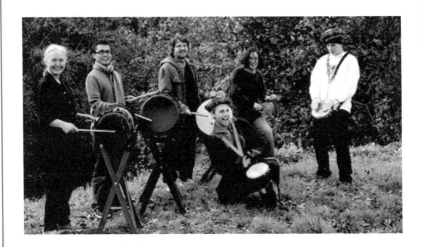

Case study 2

D originally trained as a health care professional and worked successfully for many years before an existing sight impairment deteriorated despite surgery. The termination of his employment was negotiated. After doing some project work with the then Welsh Development Agency he realised that he had developed considerable knowledge about the Disability Discrimination Act. He decided to put the knowledge to use and develop a new career and business.

D worked with the Enter DW Client Adviser to identify and develop the business idea. Contact with the mainstream business advice agency was not successful as a lot of the information and support available was not accessible to D. Consequently D started the business without exploring all the options until the Enter DW Client Adviser spent some time with him completing a basic business plan. The focus of the business was to be training and policy development around disability issues, but the planning process also identified some skills and interests not previously identified in the context of the business, notably around involvement in the arts and creative writing. Barriers to running the business were identified around administration and transport and this information was used to make an application to Access to Work for appropriate support. Following assessment and negotiation support time was agreed for administration and transport plus assistance with voice-activated and text-reading software.

The Enter DW Client Adviser introduced D to a broker who supported D with applying for and administering permitted work to allow him to develop his business and test the market whilst retaining the option of benefits should the business idea not prove viable. D's aims for the first year were to replace his benefits, an aim which happily he exceeded. D is now self-reliant for income and has developed the business to include freelance teaching in further and higher education.

Case study 3

E worked as a direct payments personal assistant, having previously worked for social services and several domiciliary care agencies. She had ambitions to set up a domiciliary care agency, not least to ensure that she could continue working whilst adapting to a deteriorating sight condition.

The Enter DW Client Adviser had previously worked for a domiciliary care agency so was able to advise on legal requirements, processes and contractual arrangements. A referral was made to the local enterprise support agency for women who provided support and training around business planning and set up. The plan was for E to initially develop the business whilst relying on her part-time wages from the personal assistant work. E was supported to make an application to Access to Work for assessment and support regarding her sight impairment.

Twelve months after starting, E's domiciliary care agency was employing 14 carers and providing support to 40 clients across three county council areas. All staff were registered for formal qualifications and one had been promoted internally to a senior position. E had finished her personal assistant work and was drawing a salary from the business. She also employed an administrator and her partner, and had moved to larger premises.

Case study 4

F had spent his working life on the production line of a local factory and had several years' experience as union shop steward. On being made redundant in his 40s with the closure of the factory he and a colleague had retrained with the aim of setting up a health and safety consultancy.

Whilst he had not been formally assessed F was aware that he probably had dyslexia which he had adapted to throughout his working life. This was now causing problems with the business as he was heavily reliant on his business partner for all administration, for example all letters and presentations had to be proofread.

F was referred to the Enter DW Client Adviser by the local enterprise information agency. After meeting and discussing the issues an application and representation was made to Access to Work for assessment and advice, with support being provided throughout the process.

The dyslexia assessment confirmed that F had dyslexia with considerable support needs, and appropriate supports were put in place. The process was affirming for F as he could finally state that his verbal reasoning skills were excellent and that there were supports for the things that he could not do so well.

Case study 5

G approached Enter at Disability Wales with ideas about setting up a transport and taxi service. He had previously worked as a specialist engineer until an accident in which he sustained head injuries resulted in several months' recuperation and rehabilitation. G had not done any detailed work developing the business idea and he was still making progress after the accident. Support provided focused on seeking practical information about the type of business whilst identifying what G wanted from work relative to what he was physically able to do.

The subsequent business planning identified that the financial outlay and running costs for the business relative to the income identified by analysis of competitors could exceed G's potential earning capacity from the hours that he could physically work. G's wife had concerns at his capacity to work at the required pace. During this process G was approached by a company with whom he had previously had contact as they were looking for somebody who knew the business who could provide admin and support on a flexible part-time basis.

Discussion identified that this was the preferred option for G who was satisfied that he had explored the potential for his business idea, a decision that was supported by G's wife.

Conclusion

The longer-term aim of the Potentia project is to develop and support the mainstream business advice services to provide support to the specific needs of different groups rather than a 'one size fits all' service. The plans are to provide training and toolkits to mainstream services to encourage a diversity of support to meet the diverse needs of entrepreneurs in setting up their own businesses.

There are lessons to be learnt by more traditional social care organisations from the way that the potential entrepreneurs are put at the centre of the process and have clear control over it. Some of the entrepreneurs and client advisers are direct payments employers and they state that there are similarities in their ability to take control and specify the services that they receive, which they can ensure are truly tailored to their personal needs in every aspect of their lives including, but not exclusively, issues relating to any impairment.

Further information can be found at:

Disability Wales
www.disabilitywales.org
www.enterdisabilitywales.co.uk/index.html

Entrepreneurship Action Plan
www.wefo.wales.gov.uk/resource/DanielJones_BusSupp4871.pdf

Objective 1 Entrepreneurship Action Plan
www.wefo.wales.gov.uk/resource/mcs_annex_f_to_paper_5.pdf

CHAPTER 6

Family Group Conferencing and 'Partnership'

James Cox

> *Doing more of the same won't work. Increasing demand, greater complexity, and rising expectations mean that the current situation is not sustainable. Tomorrow's solutions will need to engage people as active participants... Social work services do not have all the answers.*
>
> Scottish Executive (2006a, p.8)

Introduction

This chapter explores the theme of 'partnership' in those Family Group Conferences (FGCs) which are about child protection, child care planning and the welfare of children 'in need'. FGCs are a structured means of supporting family leadership in decision making. They can also promote partnership between professionals and those within the child's network who may contribute to practical planning and support. It should be noted that in Scotland FGCs are often termed 'Family Group Meetings'.

It is argued that FGC processes can be an integrated element and integrating principle within the continuum of children and families services, from prevention to permanency, and beyond permanency, to the preservation of permanent placement.

To date, FGCs have not in general been embedded within the mainstream of local authority children and families policy and services. Early UK pilot projects were set up in 1991 (Brown 2003). Subsequently local authority children and families services have become ever more tightly bound in professional and interdisciplinary procedures, particularly in relation to 'child protection'. The means to promote partnership with families have received less focus than efforts to tighten inter-agency co-operation.

Families who need considerable support in care and planning for their children should not be judged as incapable of acting in partnership unless and until they have been offered a structured and genuine opportunity to contribute in co-operation with each other and with lead professionals. FGCs can provide this opportunity and, from a child's perspective, they can also be a means of bringing reality to the injunction and title of the Scottish Child Protection Audit and Review, namely that 'It is everyone's job to make sure I'm alright' (Scottish Executive 2002).

Family Group Conference development

FGCs have been applied in diverse settings for a wide range of purpose. Burford and Hudson (2000) have provided an international overview of new directions in practice. The term 'family group conferencing' has been used internationally since the 1990s to describe structured and supported processes offered by both local authorities and voluntary agencies. The Family Rights Group introduced a clearly defined method of family group decision making into the UK in 1991. This derived from a specific model of FGC developed in New Zealand, following implementation of the New Zealand Children, Young People and Their Families Act 1989. However, some of the principles of family group conferencing have probably been an integral part of earlier forms of family group decision making in various settings, cultures and situations.

Family group conferencing practice developed in the USA from 1989, with the active encouragement of the American Humane Association. The model is now used in different forms in at least 40 US states (Merkel-Holguin, Nixon and Burford 2003). The first Australian project was set up in 1992, and through the 1990s the model was applied in Canada, Sweden, Norway, Denmark and Canada. A survey conducted in 2003–4 showed that at least 17 countries used family group conferencing across a wide range of fields, including education, mental health, justice, health, child and family welfare, communities and the workplace (Nixon *et al.* 2005). One of the findings of this survey was that 'in most cases it is practice that leads innovation and has a consequent effect on policy and law, rather than the other way around' (p.4). Although common values are identifiable across a range of setting and purpose, local politics, culture, legislation, demography and history always shape practice. Diversity of setting and of service definition are factors which make it difficult to generalise about research and evaluation findings.

In England and Wales a survey in 2001 revealed that around 38 per cent of local authorities had an FGC project (Brown 2003). By 2006 the charity Children 1st had set up 14 FGC projects in Scotland, by which time one Scottish local authority had set up an 'in-house' service. Other authorities are considering proposals. In 2006 the Family Rights Group, the Department for Education and Skills and the Welsh Assembly Government (Ashley *et al.* 2006) produced an FGC 'toolkit' to assist in FGC development and practice (available from 2007 in a Welsh version). In 2007 Children 1st launched guidance on standards and good practice on family group conferencing in Scotland.

Family Group Conference processes

In any context, FGCs are a process, not a single event. The main activities in this process are described below.

1. *Individual preparation* is offered to all potential participants. This means children, family members, in some cases significant family friends, key professionals and any advocates. At all stages the FGC coordinator retains an independence from case management, and makes it clear that an FGC is not set up as family therapy, or as an alternative to an assessment or child protection investigation. The coordinator cannot provide long-term casework. Professionals participating may need as much preparation as family members. For example, research in relation to FGCs in child protection cases (Gallagher and Jasper 2003) indicates that health visitors can feel unprepared and uncertain of their role in an FGC if they have not had adequate information about the model prior to involvement.

2. *Negotiating attendance.* In the UK FGCs are a voluntary process. Potential participants must agree the need for an FGC in order to agree a plan for a child or young person. Meetings are prepared and convened by a coordinator who is independent of case management. The coordinator does not conduct an 'assessment'. However, it is crucial that in preparation for a meeting the coordinator listens to differing family and professional perspectives. This reduces the likelihood of unhelpful

surprises in the meeting. Sometimes the process of preparation can lead to a resolution before a meeting is held.

3.   *Setting a place to meet.* When the FGC takes place, it will usually be in a neutral venue, rather than a social work office or private family flat. Participants are made welcome. Refreshment is provided. The coordinator facilitates the FGC, which will usually have three stages. These stages are for (1) introductions and information sharing, (2) private family discussion and (3) practical planning.

4.   *Meeting first stage – information sharing.* The first part of the meeting is an introduction, in which the main purposes of the meeting are confirmed, essential information is shared, and relatives have a chance to ask questions. At this stage there must be professional clarity about the limits to recommendations or decisions which could be made by the family in this meeting. Such parameters usually relate to the identified safety concerns of statutory services and to the legal situation.

5.   *Meeting second stage – private family time.* The central part of the meeting is private to the family. They have an opportunity to try and form a practical and realistic plan or set of recommendations. This part of the meeting sets FGCs apart from most other meetings attended and dominated by professionals, and efforts should be made by the coordinator to preserve this structured opportunity for the family to do business with supported independence. There are some situations where an advocate for a child or vulnerable participant may remain with the family by common agreement. There are also some situations where the family will collectively insist that the coordinator remains, for instance because of intractable and diverting conflict. In such situations, the coordinator's role is to try and ensure all parties are heard, to keep the focus on future planning, and to resist the pressure to provide solutions.

6.   *Meeting third stage – planning.* In the third and final part of the meeting, those key professionals involved rejoin the family and jointly agree the practicalities of plans and recommendations which fall within the predefined legal and safety parameters. The plan should detail how decisions should be reviewed or developed. This is often by means of planned follow-up meetings, with a view to complementing and

informing any other statutory reviews or decision-making meetings in which parents and their children may be involved.

7. *Record of agreements.* The coordinator summarises and circulates the practical agreements or disagreements reached. With the consent of participants, the record of FGC agreements can be put before the subsequent child protection case conference, a 'looked after' child review, the children's hearings or an adoption panel. Within current systems the FGC does not replace any of these other episodes. However, the FGC can provide an understanding of the family position and recommendations which are necessary for any welfare-based decision.

Decision making and Family Group Conferences

The case for an FGC could usefully and routinely be considered, for example, when a child may need:

- an integrated plan and co-operation between a range of professionals and family members
- compulsory measures
- a foster family or residential placement
- a 'child protection plan', between professionals and family members, following evidence of abuse or neglect
- long-term placement apart from birth parents
- a plan for reunification with birth family after placement in public care.

Service referral profile: An example

In one local authority service where referrals were invited at the above critical junctures (City of Edinburgh 2004), the priority problems triggering referral at the time of a first evaluation were (in order of frequency): parental drug and alcohol problems; parental mental illness; acute family conflict; child behaviour beyond parental control; domestic violence; offending by young person; physical ill health or death of parent; and other child protection concerns. The main aspirations of those referring and referred were (in order of frequency): prevention of avoidable accommodation of child (or supporting a child's return home); arrangement of complex contact or repair of loss of contact; measures to safeguard a child at home; reduction of isolation for parent and/or child; and support for change in a child's relationships in school and at home. In a preliminary and unpublished analysis, main outcomes of family meetings held were (in order of frequency): supports offered to child and family by other relatives (31%); contact agreements (31%); child looked after by relatives (20%); agreements about communication within the family (14%); and failure to reach any agreement (4%). Inevitably many referrals encompassed a combination of issues and outcomes. In this evaluation 48 per cent of families felt a clear plan had been made which was working; 6 per cent felt a plan had been made which worked for a while; and 6 per cent were not sure. Twenty-nine per cent felt the plan was not working as intended, but 53 per cent felt that communication between key parties was improved as a result of the family meeting process.

The meaning and limits of 'partnership'

In child welfare and child protection the term 'partnership' is often used loosely by professionals, as an aspirational standard for good practice in relations between professionals and service users. Partnership implies a measure of equality and agreed decision sharing between those involved. However, in almost all child care planning which involves both professionals and carers or family members there are usually both stark and subtle differences in authority, responsibility and influence between the parties involved (Hill 2000). At times FGCs may be promoted in oversimplified terms, with broad claims that can undermine the credibility of the approach. Not all families are 'their own experts'. Not all families know or can lead professionals to 'what works for them'. In reality the concept of partnership with and within families is conditional, layered and will sometimes be completely elusive. Chronic family problems are often mirrored by chronic professional 'monitoring'. However, FGCs can be a means of progressing beyond assessment and monitoring to deliberate and practical engagement.

The 1989 Children Act and 1995 Children (Scotland) Acts lead the expectation of parental involvement and responsibility for planning and decision making, with minimum intrusion, and avoidance of compulsory orders, so far as this is compatible with children's safety and welfare. Partnership in this context involves reasonable efforts to work in agreement with parents, helping them to fulfil their responsibilities. Partnership involves recognition of family, community and cultural context, strengths and weaknesses.

This is clearly no simple prescription. Social workers undertaking child protection work are usually committed to being participative with parents. However, the tension between investigation and working in partnership with the families concerned produces conflicts of interests and rights. This tension strongly affects the engagement of many families (Bell 1999). However, effective partnership between professionals and family members is rarely more necessary than in situations of continuing risk and uncertainty.

Although FGCs are intended to promote family decision-making, they do not release agencies from statutory responsibilities. FGC processes can effectively support professionals in working 'with' as well as 'for' children and their families, and can balance those professional decision-making processes which silently, by default, may remove or undermine parental and wider family responsibilities.

As with other support services, family group conferencing works best when key participants want to be involved and want the process to work. This partly depends on how the service is explained and how it is perceived. Family members tend to respond to evidence that they are being heard and respected, and if they see that the service is intended to promote their contribution to the best plan for their children. They value honesty in preparation. In common with other services, participants respond constructively to being asked what they would recommend, and what plans and services they believe would benefit the children. It is crucial that participants understand the independent role of the coordinator in relation to assessment and decision-making processes. A sense of partnership usually relates closely to the practicality of the plan which emerges. There is a shortage of long-term follow up on perceptions of FGC outcomes. Partnership may be an empty word in conferences which are called simply as a means of extracting resources from a family, as a covert assessment tool, as a rubber stamp or as a way to pressure people in to admitting certain behaviours. Coordinators should be wary of allowing conferences to be used to fit the professional plan.

Partnership: Professional expectations

They don't feel we hear them, and they think we only hear what we want to hear. Having an independent coordinator can show the family that we aren't just concerned to show social work is right. I think that's a key. (Feedback from referring social worker, 2004)

Referring social workers, highly motivated to work in partnership, can be demoralised by a sense of being driven into an adversarial role with parents in the process of protecting children. Although the principle may be implicit, the term 'partnership' does not appear in the 1989 Children Act or 1995 Children Scotland Act. Partnership is also implied in principles underlying National Standards in Scotland, though the manner of partnership is elusive in some of the detail. For example, it is a curious feature of the (Scottish) National Care Standards for Fostering and Family Placement Services that there is no section which deals with expectations of fostering services in relationship with the birth families of children placed. The Code of Ethics for the British Association of Social Workers and the Scottish Social Services Council Codes of Practice also embody values which promote partnership. However, in many instances these general expectations are not supported by local authority guidance that integrates policy and practice about the sort of interventions and services available across a spectrum of situations, to do with prevention, support, protection, reunification or permanency.

Outcomes and participant experience

Project evaluations tend to focus on the qualitative experience of participants. The research information base on the complex analysis of FGC outcomes remains slender. Although Brown (2003; Brown and Lupton 2002) has noted that there are no studies which test the FGC against other forms of decision-making process, this complaint does not weaken the case for FGCs as a process complementary to hearings, reviews and case conferences. In some cases they may be diversionary or preventative, precluding the need for compulsory processes. In others they can reduce the duration or influence the direction and outcome of compulsory measures, and in all these circumstances 'either/or' comparisons are not helpful. Within Scotland Hamilton (2005) has brought together the considerable data available from Children 1st FGC projects between 1999 and 2005 (372 meetings and 205 additional significant pieces of work from 884 referrals, involving 3866 family members). Children 1st has had a powerful endorsement of the process up to the point of the meeting, in that 91 per cent of participants offered a positive overall response to the FGC. However, here, as elsewhere, there is a gap in knowledge about outcomes.

Holland *et al.* (2003) found in a study of an independent service providing FGCs for three Welsh local authorities that almost all the family members who had experienced traditional social services planning meetings and statutory reviews preferred the experience of the FGC. In the same study, referring social workers presented a mix of value-based concepts (such as 'family empowerment' and 'hearing the voice of the child') and institutional priorities (such as 'making families take on more caring duties' and 'making families understand the seriousness of their family problems'). It was curious that, while many families saw the FGC as a means to get more help, none of the referring social workers saw the FGC as a means of getting more external help to families. Some hoped the FGC would reduce state intervention and resourcing. However, Lupton and Stevens (1997), Marsh and Crow (1998) and Smith and Hennessey (1998) found, as in Holland *et al.*'s 2003 study, that FGCs reduce unhelpful aspects of power imbalances between professionals and families. They can also moderate unhelpful power differences within families, for instance, by giving children a voice.

Meeting processes do not always go as expected, or according to plan, and even when they do they can be stressful for family members. Individual preparation, groundrules and a clear focus on the children may reduce rather than prevent surprises, conflict and other diversions, as feedback from family participants in one Scottish service revealed in 2004:

In the private time we could have our own discussions and disagreements and that was useful.

I knew how it was supposed to go, but it did not go that way.

The plan was superficial because the commitment was not there from the family.

Nothing the coordinator could have done could have taken away the anxiety about meeting.

An unexpected person turned up. That made me angry. It affected the whole meeting for me.

I think for us it was a breakthrough. It was the first time we had been able to say directly to each other what our worries were.

What we thought was the main problem turned out not to be. It was a lot of different things all rolled in to one.

The thing that made me very happy was seeing the family gather round the children and making them realise they were supported.

We got the feeling we were all on the same side.

I saw myself heard and not shut out.

It's giving people a voice that have been living in violence for years and have really been struggling. It's really been a great help.

The qualitative experience of participants is crucial, because it indicates constructive communication and allows practical joint planning. A sense of partnership is not the first experience of families if professional authority is exercised against their wishes in the protection of their children. Child protection and care planning procedures may underline the need to involve parents, but in practice many parents can often feel afraid, angry, confused and blamed. Family members significant to the children's care and protection may not know what is happening until after decisions are made. Too often, assessment and decision making is presented, defined and resourced almost exclusively by professionals. FGCs can sometimes provide an antidote to these tendencies.

Practical outcomes: examples

Most plans emerging from FGCs involve a variety of declared family intentions, offers and resources. Some happen immediately and work well, others work in part and others cannot be sustained. Where children are already subject to compulsory measures of supervision, the family make a recommendation which is then considered by the Children's Hearing. It should be recognised that in many situations there is a constructive outcome or resolution of the key issue in the preparation stage.

It may be illustrative to capture some of the central decisions from a range of different types of FGC in a local authority service:

- respite plans agreed by way of a private foster placement

- family decision *against* rehabilitation of a child from foster care to extended family

- contact arranged with extended family arranged to support permanent placement

- contact arranged between separated siblings in foster care with each other and their extended family

- an alternative to permanency plans presented by relatives who will provide respite and support to children of parent with mental health problems

- permanent care offer by a relative of separated siblings in public care

- conflict about care plan resolved between grandparents, social workers and carers

- family support offered for young person leaving residential school

- recommendation led by young person whose parents had both died: residential care rather than foster care

- 'fall back plans' made with relatives about care of child, in case of parental relapse with alcohol and drug problems

- following death of parent: there is a series of FGCs and a private fostering arrangement is assessed, supported and becomes a permanent home base, with agreed contact with extended family

- safety plans and support for young person and mother in situation of domestic violence

- agreement about risk assessment needed before any FGC (e.g. in relation to alleged sexual offences by adult)

- attention to assessment and support needs of non-resident parent with learning difficulties

- plan for assistance in tracing of parents, relatives and adopted siblings

- education and care support plans for depressed child missing school

- household agreements about rules, roles and boundaries between parents, children and relatives at a time when child might have been accommodated

- shared care and safeguards in situation of parental problem drug and alcohol use

- supported reunification plan from relative to parent.

Partnership and independence in service provision

For participants, FGC services coordinated by voluntary agencies have an obvious structural independence from the assessment, casework and decision making of local authority social work services. Voluntary agencies have already played a critical role in promoting family decision making for children, through strategic lobbying, training, good practice guidance, national practitioner networking and practical service delivery. The Family Rights Group in England and Wales and Children 1st in Scotland have been leaders in this respect. They have played an essential part in the survival and development of the approach. Barnardo's and National Children's Homes have also, in combination with the Family Rights Group, produced practice guidance (Lawrence and Wiffin 2002). Children 1st (formerly the RSSPCC) has been promoting the approach in Scotland since 1998 and, in partnership with a growing number of local authorities, they had employed 25 coordinators and a national development manager by 2006.

There is no comparative research available on the impact of structural independence on perceptions of partnership. For the one current 'in-house' service in Scotland, in the period March 2003–October 2006 (over the course of 280 referrals), there were no complaints about collusion or lack of independence. It is equally important that services are sustainable, routinely considered at key junctures and quickly accessible. For these reasons it is important that the argument for structural independence does not freeze development of in-house developments which may prove efficient for some authorities. Scottish families may benefit in future from a mixed economy of service provision.

Involvement of children

> It was important the adults heard what the children were saying. It was the most powerful part of the process. (Feedback from professional participant, 2004)

Children are too often the last people helped to understand life-changing decisions made about them by their parents or by professionals. However, professionals and families are obliged to regard children as partners. Under the Children (Scotland) Act 1995 a person reaching any major decision in fulfilment of parental responsibilities, or acting as a carer, or a person who is exercising a parental right or giving consent, must have regard 'so far as is practicable' to the views of the child (if the child wishes to express them), taking account of the child's age and maturity. The duties of local authorities to 'looked after' children are set out in s17(3) and to children who may be accommodated, under s25.5. The views and feelings of children must be considered in a wide range of circumstances (Marshall *et al.* 2002). Children are persons, and in the language of the 1998 Human Rights Act they possess Convention Rights. FGCs are a means of applying this central principle of the UN Convention on Rights of the Child (UNCRC) and the Children (Scotland) Act 1995. UNCRC stipulates that children's views will be considered and taken into account in all matters that affect them. It is current Scottish Executive policy to reflect the articles of the Convention in all changes and developments affecting children. Family group conferencing is one of those services which may be considered as a means of supporting children's involvement in decision making.

Children and young people can contribute to the planning of an FGC and may be present throughout or for part of a meeting. However, there are a variety of ways in which children can contribute their views and feelings. Some choose to send a letter to a FGC. Others prefer to be represented by a trusted adult. Most children old and confident enough to articulate their hopes, fears and ideas will be able to contribute directly (Hamilton 2005; Lupton and Stevens 1997; Marsh and Crow 1998), or with the help of a non-family member acting as an advocate (Dalrymple 2002). An FGC coordinator will in almost all circumstances make efforts to hear the child in preparation for a meeting and will involve them directly in all or part of a meeting, as appropriate to the circumstances, and taking into account the views of those who know the child best and have key responsibilities for the child's care. However, there are some circumstances in which to involve the child would traumatise them further, or place them in a situation of intolerable anxiety or divided loyalties.

The communication skills of the professionals involved are crucial to the child's effective participation. Although there is no research currently on the specific participation of disabled children in FGCs, Cavet and Sloper (2004) have produced a relevant review of literature about the participation of disabled children in decisions made about their lives.

As an overarching principle, all decisions made in partnership or otherwise are subject to the welfare principle. Guidance on the UN Convention on Rights of the Child states that a partnership approach has as its goal the best interests of the child.

The meaning of 'family'

'Working in partnership with families' is an aspiration additionally complicated by the diffuse meaning of 'family' in law, to professionals, and in the varied experience of those within their margins. In the context of FGC development reference is inevitably made to New Zealand, where minority Maori social structures, traditions and values apparently provided a compact incentive to respect the co-operative strength of culturally accepted decision-making processes. Although FGC principles are transferable to a range of cultural settings, it could be argued that there is no similar motivational coherence in the complex of cultures and disparate family structures which must be served by social services in the UK.

The term 'family', in the context of FGCs, refers both to blood relatives and to non-related significant family friends or neighbours. Even without this extended definition, the term 'family' contains a bewildering diversity of meaning. There is no recognised legal entity in UK legislation called 'the family'. In contrast, the Irish Constitution in Article 41.1.1 explicitly confers rights on the family. Many children caught up in child welfare processes have not been nurtured and held in their development by a family 'unit' of reliable definition. They may have tenuous connections with the shards of several families, perhaps including non-relative private or public foster carers. Relatives who appear closely related on a professionally constructed 'genogram' may rarely have met each other. These relatives may have no common purpose or view in relation to the child's interests. They may not wish to be in a room together. There is no research to suggest that family decision making about children tends to be democratic. On the contrary, the experience and views of significant family members are often unknown to or ignored by decision makers within each family. Overall, coordinators are concerned to identify and engage with those who care about the child and may be in a position to help.

Engaging with fathers

Fathers can be marginalised or ignored, particularly in situations where children are known to social and health services because of abuse or neglect (Daniel and Taylor 2001). While underlining the need for careful risk assessment, Daniel and Taylor offer practical and theoretical guidance, supported by case examples and service initiatives. Men who have been excluded from their children's lives can be encouraged as fathers while challenging, if necessary, unhelpful aspects of their masculinity. This is valuable contextual reading for coordinators who are likely to be exploring the potential inclusion of absent parents in FGC processes.

Competing rights in partnership

Tensions between the rights of parents and those of children or other family members further complicate the exercise of partnership. At times the wishes and interests of family members and of children involved are congruent, and at times they are in conflict. FGCs offer one way of openly identifying and attempting to reconcile these tensions within a practical plan. Social workers, Safeguarders in the children's hearings and court-appointed curators have roles in the representation of children's best interests. Effective FGC processes do not replace various forms of assessment, reporting and representation. They are often a useful connection between assessment and resolution, by means of a plan which, by family agreement, puts the child's interests first. However, the Scottish Executive (2004) issued a Children's Charter and national framework for standards in child protection which in many instances could be strongly supported by the FGC approach.

Coordinating FGCs: Challenges and requirements

There are a range of common challenges and dilemmas that will be familiar to most coordinators and referring social workers. For the purposes of an FGC, it can be hard to resolve who finally defines which people are 'the family'. It is normal to hear a range of perceptions about who is significant, who may be harmful, or even about which relatives exist. Professionals may only partially understand how decisions are made within a family. There may be suspicions that family group decision making is constrained by bullying or secrecy in a way that cannot be proven or controlled. In situations of serious risk, it seems reasonable to question if family group conferencing should be offered if there is no relative who has ever recognised or effectively protected the child's needs.

Where children have been subject to serious deprivation and abuse, their involvement in decision making should be handled in a way that is right for their age, stage, understanding and experience. When there are essential gaps in professional knowledge about historical risk to children, FGCs can accentuate existing risks by presenting plans, disguise gaps in assessment and even discourage external support.

Common ingredients in children and families social work include parental isolation, domestic violence and family decision making steered by addiction. In some circumstances it may be impossible or destructive to convene a meeting of all significant relatives. At other times it may be in the children's interests if an adapted service is offered, where the independent coordinator applies the key principles and structure to a meeting or series of meetings with key individuals within the family.

In situations of high and chronic risk it remains likely that professionals will have a leading hand in protective decision making, and will not simply 'go with the family plan', but will consider carefully whether new family proposals offer adequate safeguards. Plans may have to be tested out step by step and commitment to sustaining them may be transitory.

There is little international consensus about the job specification, role and status for FGC coordinators. Not all projects require independent coordinators. Not all projects require coordinators to be social work qualified. The way in which the coordinator applies their own value base will have an impact on outcome and on participants' perception of partnership. Good practice guidance on the Family Rights Group website insists that the coordinator should reflect the race and culture of the family and share the same first language. This is not easy to achieve, and relevant consultation should be sought where cross-cultural services are provided. The process should be held in the family's first language with, where necessary, the professionals using interpreters.

As a minimum coordinators require a sound understanding of statutory processes, and the ways in which they can be complemented rather than replaced by FGCs. They also require a realistic appreciation of circumstances or stages where the model cannot be applied and a child-centred and sometimes flexible approach to application of FGC principles.

Legal mandate and strategic leadership

In contrast to New Zealand, Australia, the Republic of Ireland and Sweden, there has been no UK legislation defining or requiring family group conferencing at times of critical statutory child care decision making about children. Family group conferencing projects are usually small scale and under intense pressure to justify their existence in terms of numbers of referrals and positive outcomes. Doolan (2002) argues that there is a need for a prescriptive legal mandate for family group conferencing, as well as clear expectations in standards, procedures and guidelines on good practice. He has witnessed many projects struggling inefficiently with existing systems, professional assumptions, procedures and organisational protocols. With the exception of a limited statement by the Department of Health in 1999 (p.78), which described the conference process as a 'positive option for planning services for children and families', there has been no central government guidance in England or in Scotland encouraging standard consideration of family group conferencing at key junctures in child care planning.

However, FGCs were promoted and endorsed by guidance issued by the National Assembly for Wales (2000 and 2001). This guidance states that FGCs should not be used as an alternative to Child Protection Case Conferences, but are a useful way of furthering child protection plans and working more effectively in partnership with the families of children 'in need'. In the one local authority which has an in-house service, over the period 2003–5, most families have responded well to the voluntary opportunity to work together. Others who have not engaged might possibly have responded if they had been required in law to take part in FGC processes in prescribed circumstances. It is difficult to generalise about the potential advantage of a legal mandate on the basis of current research. FGCs are unlikely to be incorporated in Scottish legislation over the next five years (as there are no proposals to this effect under consideration). However, it would lend authority and incentive to organisational developments if consideration of FGCs at critical episodes in decision making was encouraged in guidance on current revision to Scottish adoption and fostering regulations and within Scottish national fostering and kinship care strategies (Scottish Executive 2006c).

Nixon and Burford's international survey in 2005 found that there is often a stress between the need for flexibility of practice, and the need for regulation to sustain practice. Most new projects struggle to get conferencing integrated with mainstream services and procedures, and usually a significant commitment in funding, management support and policy (if not law) is needed to sustain successful conferencing.

Development of this form of partnership across the UK has relied on the local persistence and values of individual managers and practitioners. The values and practice of individual referring professionals on the ground also determine the extent to which the model is used in practice and the way in which it is used to promote partnership (Sundell 2000).

In Scotland central government leadership is likely to be critical to the development of this form of partnership. The Report of the Child Protection Audit and Review (Scottish Executive 2002) bluntly categorised systemic barriers to partnership in Scotland. A driving theme in the Report is a need for 'greater coherence' in children's services. Three main aspects of child protection – protection services, criminal justice and children's hearings – are not well aligned. Within separated specialisms professionals struggle to respond to children's needs in a holistic way. The Audit specifically recommended that the interface between children's services and the hearing systems needs to be improved because of cumbersome, lengthy, partial and often duplicated processes, which frequently do not enhance children's safety or provide coherent, individualised support plans for their families in keeping the children safe. FGCs are a means of addressing the families' experience of this systemic and professional disintegration. However, this can only occur if its principles are politically understood and promoted, and if each service is practically led and supported by those who direct local statutory services.

Extraordinary Lives is the title of the Social Work Inspection Agency's 2006 review of 'looked after' children in Scotland. The theme of partnership with children and families recurs frequently, especially with regard to support of kinship care arrangements, though specific recommendations are not made about FGC development.

Since April 1997, Scottish local authorities have been required to publish plans for 'relevant services' for children (1995 Act, s19, and Plans for Services for Children Directions 1996). This should reasonably include information about the option of FGCs in relation to prevention, protection, support and permanency. Consistent and effective front-line partnership must be underpinned by integrated policies, strategies and service guidelines, and cannot be sustained by isolated initiatives.

To date, the review of the children's hearings system in Scotland (Scottish Executive 2005) has consulted upon but not publicly represented ways in which family group conferencing could complement the hearings system. Many of the intentions within the *Getting It Right for Every Child Implementation Plan* (Scottish Executive 2006b, p.5), guidance on planning for children (Scottish Executive 2007) and the draft Children's Services (Scotland) Bill would be well supported by family group conferencing services.

Assessment, risk and Family Group Conferences

FGC coordinators do not conduct assessments, although they may unearth evidence of risk. Safe FGC processes are therefore dependent on the adequacy of preceding and sometimes of subsequent risk assessments (for example, when assessments needed before a recommended family plan can be agreed). FGC services attempt to promote partnership, but as this partnership is compatible with children's safety and welfare, it is argued that coordinators should also have a firm stance or precondition in relation to some forms of identified risk. If this does not happen the FGC process is more likely to lead to the setting up of plans which disguise or accentuate existing dangers.

For instance, where there is a background of family violence and an expectation that the FGC will resolve residence and contact issues, it is recommended that an FGC should not proceed unless there is:

- full acknowledgement of the violence by the perpetrator
- acceptance of responsibility for the violence
- acceptance of the likely impact of the violence
- evidence of a wish to make reparation to the child and others in the household who have been affected by the violence
- evidence of ability to sustain promises or commitments.

These would be among the necessary considerations in legal decisions about contact arrangements in situations of domestic violence (Butler-Sloss, Thorpe and Waller 2000) and in any social work assessment (Calder 2005). There may be a range of other risk factors and considerations which are not known at the point of referral. Essential elements of FGC processes in situations of domestic violence are illustrated by Burford and Hudson (2000, Chapter 16). In the UK the Dove Daybreak Project in Hampshire is an example of a service which specialises in FGC work in situations of domestic violence. It is jointly funded between police, health and social services projects. Their ethos is that 'violence against any member of the family is violence against the entire family, hitting at its very heart'. The service assumes that widening the circle around the family safeguards the child and adult members (Powney 2004). Feedback from family members at the Dove Project sheds light on the value of the FGC process. For example:

> The meeting made us closer. The problem was brought out into the open. It was easier to deal with because there was more help. (Young mother)

> The plan makes a difference. It stops us fighting. (Young mother)

> It was a different way of airing things that had been locked up. (Young person)

The victim has re-established family links and this makes her feel safer. (Professional participant)

These considerations and potential advantages translate to FGCs where there are other or additional forms of risk (such as drug use or sexual abuse). The aim would be to ensure that key stakeholders inside or outside the family are mobilised to work on the issue. The coordinator should ensure there are strategies in place to protect participants. Sufficient information, support and privacy must be provided in the meeting to allow the family group to form a sound plan. Where plans evidently promote the safety and welfare of the child and adult family members the plan should be approved. Resources should be authorised to support the plan, and limits to resources should be clarified in advance. Any plan which emerges from a family meeting should clarify how progress can be reviewed. An essential principle is to support and sustain community and family partnerships that safeguard the child and adult survivors.

Although coordinators do not conduct assessments, it is dishonest to pretend that an FGC will not enhance crucial elements of social work assessment. After all, the process often illustrates the potential for co-operation with and within the family. However, family group conferencing cannot replace analysis of and work with the causes of risk. In situations of known or suspected risk to children, family group meetings must be preceded by an assessment which integrates information about the child and family history held by key professionals across disciplines.

Family Group Conferences and effective child protection

There has been a significant increase in the number of child protection orders taken in Scotland in the period from 1999 to 2005 (Francis, McGhee and Mordaunt 2006). The Report of the Child Protection Audit and Review (Scottish Executive 2002) listed those features of services which are known to have contributed to the protection of children who have been abused or neglected. Effective services incorporate preventative strategies, connecting provision of support to the family and to the child. Specifically they should build on community and family strengths, and 'be trusted by children and young people to act in their best interests'. They should be easy to access and simple to understand, and offer help as and when it is needed, in the process treating children and parents with respect. They should act promptly and involve improving inter-agency work. Finally, successful services are tailored to match children's needs. This list of features is embodied in FGC principles. However, FGCs were not a service option mentioned by the above-mentioned 2002 Scottish Executive Report.

Marsh and Crow's study (1998, Table 8.6) found that, in the view of professionals involved and from an analysis of child protection register data, children were comparatively well protected by plans made and there was no increase in child protection concerns post-FGC. Brown and Lupton (2002) attempted a rigorous evaluation of FGCs in child protection in a study in a rural county in south-west England. This involved ten children and families fieldwork teams and two child health teams. They found that professionals struggled to accept shared decision making with family members, and that existing statutory child protection procedures leave very little room for FGCs to occur. For this reason some family members were confused about the remit and scope of their own meeting. Some family members did not wish to share their problems with the wider family. It was significant that, despite having an FGC service in operation for ten years in this authority, the model had not become embedded in policy, guidelines and managerial thinking, and was therefore only evident in patches of good practice. However, Brown and Lupton noted that FGCs have a positive role in tackling emotional abuse and neglect cases, in development of child protection plans and resolving contentious residence issues. Over the course of a nine-month mapping exercise Brown and Lupton concluded that FGC services appeared to make a lasting and positive difference.

Effective family support

The characteristics of effective family support are also well researched (Research in Practice 2005). They include early intervention; targeted support, where families understand the aims of services; support which uses and builds on strengths while actively tackling the main problems and vulnerabilities; and a whole family approach, which considers how services and plans should fit together rather than considering problems in isolation (Scottish Executive 2003). These findings could usefully be applied to the early consideration of FGCs and applied to strategic resourcing of plans which emerge from FGCs.

Following the death of the privately fostered child Victoria Climbié, the report of Lord Laming's Inquiry advised against dislocating the protection of children from the wider support of their families (Laming 2003). The needs of the child and the support needs of their family are often inseparable. This integral connection can be sundered by the way we often specialise and segregate investigative and support services, and by the way the role of the 'child's social worker' may be interpreted by the worker or perceived by the family. FGCs may assist in the reconnection of assessment and safety parameters with support plans which family members can understand, and by producing plans which support gaps in family care with agreed external resources. Planning reunification with birth family for a child in public care (Biehal 2006) requires the sort of careful planning with families for which this vehicle is well suited.

FGCs contribute to planning and change, but they are obviously not a self-contained solution. As one family member put it, 'Things are moving forward, but it's not all to do with the meeting.'

Permanency, partnership and Family Group Conferences

FGCs can complement and shape intensive, time-limited efforts towards reha-bilitation, and 'parallel' or 'concurrent' planning. Children 1st have given one account of how FGC processes can be applied in adoption and permanency processes (Gill, Higginson and Napier 2003). However, there is no research base for FGCs and permanency in Scotland. Impending reform in adoption and fostering legislation is likely to enhance rather than limit the potential role of FGCs, because there is likely to be a more flexible range of legal and practical possibilities for partnership in the sharing of parental responsibilities (Scottish Executive/Cox 2005).

FGC processes can be of considerable assistance under current adoption regulations and National Standards, for example, in demonstrated consider-ation of:

- family composition, circumstances and views, including those of siblings

- alternatives to adoption or long-term foster care

- contact arrangements which will promote the child's security and key relationships

- support plans for children placed and their carers (e.g. in terms of respite).

The paramount consideration for adoption panels is the child's welfare throughout life. Life-long identity and relationship issues must be considered. FGCs are a means of ensuring families have a chance to hear, digest and perhaps oppose the local authority assessment and plan. Views and options within the extended family are explored and represented. The outcome can be recorded. Even if no agreement is reached or safe alternatives identified, the reasoning and record could be valuable to the child in future.

Partnership where children are not defined as 'looked after'

Statutory reviews for 'looked after' children bring some structure to decision making that involves parents, children and relevant services. However, Morris (2005) describes how some categories of children 'in need' as defined by the 1989 and 1995 Acts may receive a less integrated and consultative service, in terms of local authority efforts to work in partnership with those jointly responsible for their care and protection. For example, children with disabilities are not often defined as 'looked after', when they are placed out of their home authority in residential special schools (SEN Regional Partnerships 2005, p.40). Many have complex needs, including emotional and behavioural problems. Abbott, Morris and Ward (2001, p.26) found that the feelings of such children and the circumstances of their families are not often known to decision makers. Few of these children wish to be placed away from home. Many parents of these children speak of a lack of understanding and lack of coordinated assistance from education and social services to look at alternatives or connected child welfare issues. Families in these circumstances can feel uncertain about what is right for their child, and powerless in the face of decisions taken by distant experts or resource gatekeepers who do not know them or their child. Family group conferencing is congruent with Scottish Office guidance on the 1995 Act (Scottish Office 1997, Vol. 1, Ch. 6, paras 18–25). In these circumstances, FGCs could assist in linking strengths, wishes and concerns within the family with best information about resources and options.

Kinship care and partnership

FGCs can be helpful in the planning and support of kinship care placements, at a time when, across the UK, kinship placements are increasing as a proportion of all foster placements and as a proportion of all children 'looked after' (Broad and Skinner 2005; Department of Health 2001, Table iv, p.23; Hunt 2003). In Scotland, as elsewhere in the UK, there is considerable variation between and sometimes within authorities on assessment, training, support and remuneration of carers. The Family Rights Group (Doolan, Nixon and Lawrence 2004) and the British Association for Adoption and Fostering (2003) have usefully contributed to debate on kinship care research, policy and practice. Scottish research on kinship placements in the context of problem drug use (Barnard 2003) has also provided a useful cautionary note.

In Scotland there is a lack of reliable information about types and numbers of placement with relatives and friends, and a lack of a consistent framework for assessment, support and remuneration. Most children are not formally 'placed' and many are unknown to local authorities. However, relatives and friends care for many 'looked after' children in Scotland. Children in 'immediate placement' also fall within the scope of the public fostering service (which must be inspected by the Care Commission). A small minority of relative and friend carers are approved as public foster carers. National Care Standards for Fostering and Family Placement do not mention relative carers (or private foster carers, some of whom may be distant relatives).

It would be helpful to have nationally defined general principles, underpinned by Scottish law and European Human Rights legislation, which cover the range of kinship care placements. The Association of Directors of Social Work has gone some way to encapsulating principles (ADSW/TFN Scotland 2003) which support and can be supported by FGC services, recommending that:

- It is the right of every child to have their family and friends explored as carers if they need to leave the care of their parents.

- Any arrangement for care by family or friend must be in the best interests of the child, and safety of the child in any assessment of family or friend as carer must be paramount.

- The wider network of family and friends should be explored before a local authority offers care.

- Support to a family or friend placement should be available when needed. Financing needs to be based on the needs of the child and the impact of providing care on the carers.

- A child's needs for family and friend carers should take precedence over the wishes of a parent to exclude the family from care.

Partnership where care arrangements are private

> I think the situation at home would have got so I would have lost contact with him altogether and that would have been severe for my other children. (Feedback on FGC processes from mother of one privately fostered teenager)

There is a comparative lack of attention accorded by local authorities to many children 'in need' or at risk who are living in private fostering arrangements (Holman 2002; Morris 2005; Philpot 2001). It is beyond the scope of this chapter to review the context, reasons and possible systemic remedies for this pattern. FGC processes can identify private fostering arrangements that are previously unknown and other potential private fostering arrangements that offer positive respite and support. FGC processes can lead to the investigation and approval of positive arrangements, or the review and supported improvement of placements that are concerning.

Family Group Conferences and limitations to brief intervention

> Obviously we did not agree properly at the end or we were not being honest with each other. It might take a few more meetings to get to that (Participant family member, evaluation of pilot service 2004)

Short-term plans emerging from family group conferencing may help reduce friction and resolve immediate crises. However, it is unusual for one FGC to make lasting change within families with multiple, long-term problems. In such situations support packages may need to be long term. A sequence of FGCs may be offered to review progress, as appropriate in each situation.

In situations of sustained and serious failure to meet children's needs, it is likely that no single method of intervention is likely to be sufficient. Practical and therapeutic help may need to be carefully coordinated, by a small core of individuals. Significant and purposeful relationships between a few key practitioners and the family are often the key to positive change.

Family group conferencing can complement and shape long-term work with families. In the absence of sustained, targeted work, families and their children may repeatedly present with the same unresolved difficulties. Although long-term work is often negatively associated with the idea of 'dependency' in the early stages of such work, families with complex needs may well need to rely heavily on individual professionals. They may well need to develop an understanding and trust in this collaborative relationship. Contracts, goal setting and reviews are standard approaches to ensuring purposeful, safe and efficient work. Family group conferencing can complement and inform various reviews and decision making integral to long-term planning and packages of care. It can allow family members to gain a sense of control over their lives, and to experience collective efforts to meet the needs of their children.

Summary

The *Report on the 21st Century Review of Social Work in Scotland* recommends that services should build on the capacity and strengths of individuals, families and communities (Scottish Executive 2006a, p.91). FGC services are a vehicle which can promote partnership in a practical manner, for example, through:

- sharing family and professional understanding of the child's needs, and the role of statutory agencies

- identifying strengths, risks and opportunities with the family network

- exploring what would be involved to make alternative care options viable and sustainable

- ensuring fractured family groups have a structured opportunity to work together with each other and with other agencies

- ensuring families have a chance to discuss and clarify professional assessments and actions

- ensuring children and separated siblings have a voice that is heard or represented in a way that is sensitive to their abilities and circumstances.

Access to such services in Scotland currently depends upon the success and scale of local projects and local service agreements. There is scope for parallel policy development in a wide range of context including housing, education and youth justice. FGC principles rather than FGC projects have the potential to bring integration and balance to the continuum of services for children and families, for instance, in prevention, respite, child protection planning, reunification, shared and kinship care arrangements, contact planning and permanency. Central government has a potential role to play in support of research and policy developments and in provision of good practice guidance.

Local projects are less likely to be effective if local authorities do not integrate FGC services and principles within their own policies and procedures.

Note

Family group conferencing as 'restorative justice' is a parallel development beyond the scope of this chapter (McCold and Wachtel 2003). Brief guidance on recommended practice in Scotland can be found at www.restorativejusticescotland.org.uk/ practices.htm.

References

Abbott, D., Morris, J. and Ward, L. (2001) *The Best Place to Be? Policy, Practice and the Experiences of Residential School Placements for Disabled Children.* York: Joseph Rowntree Foundation/York Publishing Services

Ashley, C., Holton, L., Horan, H. and Wiffin, J. (2006) *Family Group Conference Toolkit – A Practice Guide for Setting Up and Running an FGC Service.* London: Family Rights Group, Department for Education and Skills and the Welsh Assembly Government.

ADSW/TFN Scotland (2003) *Family and Friends as Carers.* Report for the Association of Directors of Social Work Working Group. Edinburgh: ADSW/TFN Scotland.

Barnard, M. (2003) 'Between a rock and a hard place: the role of relatives in protecting children from the effects of parental drug problems.' *Journal of Child and Family Social Work 8,* 291–299.

Bell, M. (1999) 'Working in partnership in child protection: the conflicts.' *British Journal of Social Work 29,* 3, 437–455.

Biehal, N. (2006) *Reuniting Looked After Children with their Families.* Rowntree Foundation Research Findings. www.jrf.org.uk/knowledge/findings/socialpolicy/pdf/ 0056.pdf, accessed on 28 September 2007.

British Association for Adoption and Fostering (2003) *Every Child Matters – Consultation Response.* www.baaf.org.uk/res/consultations/ consultresponse_ecm.pdf, accessed on 28 September 2007.

Broad, B. and Skinner, A. (2005) *Relative Benefits: Placing Children in Kinship Care.* BAAF good practice guide. London: British Association for Adoption and Fostering.

Brown, L. (2003) 'Mainstream or margin? The current use of family group conferences in child welfare practice in the UK.' *Journal of Child and Family Social Work 8,* 331–340.

Brown, L. and Lupton, C. (2002) *The Role of Family Group Conferences in Child Protection.* Wiltshire County Council/University of Bath/Nuffield Foundation/Centre for Evidence Based Social Services. Bath: University of Bath.

Burford, G. and Hudson, J. (2000) *Family Group Conferencing: New Directions in Community Centred Child and Family Practice.* New York, NY: De Gruyter.

Butler-Sloss, E., Thorpe, P. and Waller, I. (2000) *Re L; Re V; Re M; and Re H (Contact: Domestic Violence).* Court of Appeal, 19 June. *Family Law Review* 334.

Calder, M. (2005) *Children Living with Domestic Violence.* Lyme Regis: Russell House.

Cavet, J. and Sloper, P. (2004) 'Participation of disabled children in individual decisions about their lives and in public decisions about service development.' *Children and Society 18,* 278–290.

Children's Services (Scotland) Bill (draft). www.scotland.gov.uk/childrensservicesbill, accessed on 15 June 2007.

City of Edinburgh (2004) *Participant Views of Family Group Meetings 2003–4: Key Findings.* Social Work Business Support Services, Research and Information Team. Unpublished council report.

Dalrymple, J. (2002) 'Family group conferences and youth advocacy: participation of children and young people in family decision making.' *European Journal of Social Work 5,* 3, 287–299.

Daniel, B. and Taylor, J. (2001) *Engaging with Fathers: Practice Issues for Health and Social Care.* London: Jessica Kingsley Publishers.

Department of Health (1999) *Working Together to Safeguard Children.* London: The Stationery Office. www.dh.gov.uk/prod_consum_dh/ groups/dh_digitalassets/@dh/ @en/documents/digitalasset/dh_4075824.pdf, accessed on 28 September 2007.

Department of Health (2001) *Children 'Looked After' by Local Authorities, Year Ending 31 March 2000.* London: Department of Health.

Doolan, M. (2002) 'Family Group Conferences and Social Work: Some Observations about the United Kingdom and New Zealand.' Conference paper presented at Family Rights Group Conference, Manchester: Building on Strength: International Perspectives on Family Group Conferences, September 2002.

Doolan, M., Nixon, P. and Lawrence, P. (2004) *Growing Up in the Care of Relatives and Friends.* London: Family Rights Group.

Family Rights Group website: www.frg.org.uk

Francis, J., McGhee, J. and Mordaunt, E. (2006) *Protecting Children in Scotland: Risk Assessment and Interagency Collaboration in the Use of Child Protection Orders.* Scottish Executive Social Research 2006, School of Social and Political Studies, University of Edinburgh. www.scotland.gov.uk/Resource/Doc/923/0038163.pdf, accessed on 15 June 2007.

Gallagher, F. and Jasper, M. (2003) 'Health Visitors' experiences of Family Group Conferences in relation to child protection planning: a phenomenological study.' *Journal of Nursing Management 11,* 377–386.

Gill, H., Higginson, L. and Napier, H. (2003) 'Family Group Conferences in permanency planning.' *Adoption and Fostering 27,* 2, 53–63.

Hamilton, A. (2005) *Releasing the Power of the Family: Children 1st and Family Group Conference Services in Scotland 1999–2005.* Edinburgh: Children 1st.

Hill, M. (2000) 'Partnership reviewed. Words of caution, words of encouragement.' *Adoption and Fostering 24,* 3, 56–68.

Holland, S., O'Neill, S., Scourfield, J. and Pithouse, A. (2003) *Outcomes in Family Group Conferences for Children on the Brink of Care: A Study of Child and Family Participation.* Report for the Welsh Office for Research and Development in Health and Social Care. Cardiff: University of Cardiff.

Holman, B. (2002) *The Unknown Fostering: A Study of Private Practice.* Dorset: Russell House Publishing.

Hunt, J. (2003) *Family and Friends Carers.* Scoping paper for the Department of Health. www.doh.gov.uk/carers/familyandfriends.htm., accessed on 28 September 2007.

Laming, Lord (2003) *The Victoria Climbié Inquiry. Report of an Inquiry by Lord Laming.* CM 5730. Norwich: Stationery Office.

Lawrence, P. and Wiffin, J. (2002) *Family Group Conferences: Principles and Practice Guidance.* Ilford: Barnardo's/Family Rights Group/NCH.

Lupton, C. and Stevens, M. (1997) *Family Outcomes: Following through on Family Group Conferences.* SSRIU Report No.34. Portsmouth: University of Portsmouth.

Marsh, P. and Crow, G. (1998) *Family Group Conferences in Child Welfare.* Oxford: Blackwell.

Marshall, K., Tisdall, M., Cleland, A. and Plumtree, A. (2002) *'Voice of the Child' under the Children (Scotland) Act 1995: Volume 1 – Mapping Paper.* Edinburgh: Scottish Executive Central Research Unit.

McCold, P. and Wachtel, T. (2003) 'Theory of Restorative Justice.' Paper presented at the XIII World Congress of Criminology, 10–15 August, Rio de Janeiro. www.realjustice.org/library/paradigm.html, accessed on 15 June 2007.

Merkel-Holguin, L., Nixon, P. and Burford, G. (2003) 'Learning with families: a synopsis of FGDM research and evaluation in child welfare.' *Protecting Children 18*, 1–2 , 2–11 , Denver: American Humane. www.frg.org.uk/pdfs/Learning%20With%20 Families%20Report.pdf, accessed on 28 September 2007.

Morris, J. (2005) *Children on the Edge of Care: Human Rights and the Children Act.* York: York Publishing Services.

National Assembly for Wales (2000) *Working Together to Safeguard Children.* Cardiff: National Assembly for Wales.

National Assembly for Wales (2001) *Framework for Assessment of Children 'In Need' and their Families.* Cardiff: National Assembly for Wales.

Nixon, P., Burford, G., Quinn, A. and Edelbaum, J. (2005) *A Survey of International Practices, Policy and Research on Family Group Conferencing and Related Practices.* American Humane Association. www.americanhumane.org/site/DocServer/ FGDM_www_survey.pdf?docID=2841, accessed on 28 September 2007.

Philpot, T. (2001) *A Very Private Practice: An Investigation into Private Fostering.* London: BAAF.

Powney, A. (2004) 'The Daybreak Dove Project.' *Family Rights Group Newsletter,* Spring.

Research in Practice (2005) Quality Protects Research Briefing No. 10: 'Understanding and Working with Neglect' and Quality Protects Research Briefing No. 11: 'Supporting Families.' www.rip.org.uk/publications/researchbriefings.asp, accessed on 15 June 2007.

Scottish Executive (2002) *'It Is Everyone's Job to Make Sure I'm Alright.' Report of the Child Protection Audit and Review.* Edinburgh: Scottish Executive.

Scottish Executive (2003) *'Growing Support': Review of Services for Vulnerable Families with Young Children.* Edinburgh: Stationery Office. www.scotland.gov.uk/Publications/ 2003/01/15814/13977, accessed on 15 June 2007.

Scottish Executive (2004) *National Framework for Standards in Child Protection.* www.scotland.gov.uk/Publications/2004/03/19102/34603, accessed on 15 June 2007

Scottish Executive (2005) *'Getting it Right for Every Child': Consultation on the Review of the Children's Hearings System.* Edinburgh: Scottish Executive.

Scottish Executive (2006a) *Changing Lives: Report of the 21st Century Social Work Review.* www.scotland.gov.uk/Publications/2006/02/02094408/0, accessed on 15 June 2007.

Scottish Executive (2006b) 'Getting It Right for Every Child: Implementation Plan' and draft Children's Services (Scotland) Bill for consultation 20.12.06. www.scotland.gov.uk/childrensservicesbill, accessed on 15 June 2007.

Scottish Executive (2006c) *National Fostering and Kinship Care Strategy: Consultation.* Edinburgh: Scottish Executive. www.scotland.gov.uk/Publications/ 2006/12/07091551/2, accessed on 15 June 2007.

Scottish Executive (2007) *Guidance on the Child or Young Person's Plan.* Edinburgh: Scottish Executive.

Scottish Executive/Cox, G. (2005) *Adoption: Better Choices for Our Children.* The report of the Adoption Policy Review Group. Edinburgh: Scottish Executive. www.scotland.gov.uk/Publications/2005/06/27140607/06107, accessed on 15 June 2007.

Scottish Office (1997) *Social Work Services Group: Guidance on the Children (Scotland) Act 1995 (Vol. 1, Ch. 6, paras 18–25).* Edinburgh: Scottish Office.

SEN Regional Partnerships (2005) *Analysis of Out of Authority Placements.* www.teachernet.gov.uk/docbank/index.cfm?id=7154, accessed on 28 September 2007.

Smith, L. and Hennessey, J. (1998) *Making a Difference. Essex Family Group Conference Project: Research Findings and Practice Issues.* Chelmsford: Essex County Council Social Services Department.

Social Work Inspection Agency (2006) *Extraordinary Lives. Creating a Positive Future for Looked After Children and Young People in Scotland.* Edinburgh: SWIA.

Sundell, K. (2000) 'Family Group Conferences in Sweden.' In G. Burford and J. Hudson (eds) *Family Group Conferencing: New Directions in Community Centred Child and Family Practice.* New York, NY: De Gruyter.

CHAPTER 7

Person-Centred Planning as Co-Production

Steve Coulson

The concept of co-production in human services might initially provoke a sceptical chuckle. The ideas of production and consumption are inextricably linked and the image of the social care 'consumer' gamely trying to find out how to return their unsatisfactory respite or day care package speaks for itself. The poor outcomes of many human services are often attributed to a lack of resources or to inflexibility and bureaucratic inertia. The implication is that interventions, though ineffectual, are fundamentally benign and well meaning. McKnight (1995) highlights the stark reality that human services may have a more malign and damaging impact on individuals and communities in the long term and goes as far as to suggest that 'competent communities have been invaded, captured and colonized by professional services'. In this context, the idea of co-production has particular relevance. Person-centred planning, rooted in a philosophy of partnership and equality, can be genuinely empowering and useful to hitherto excluded people.

In this chapter, the key ideas underpinning person-centred planning are outlined before considering how they might best support a co-productive approach. Evidence is then provided of its effectiveness from work undertaken in Scotland, followed by an examination of some of the limitations of person-centred planning in current conditions.

What is person-centred planning?

Falvey *et al.* (2003, p.68) describe person-centred planning as: 'A constellation of tools developed to help a person or a family who want to make a purposeful and meaningful change in their life.' The phrase conjures up an inspiring image of sights set firmly on a horizon of infinite possibilities but also suggests an approach which is diverse, flexible and creative. At its very best, person-centred planning operates in this way.

However, person-centred planning is only a means to an end. The aim is inclusion, by which we mean individuals leading good and full lives in ordinary and extraordinary ways, making a genuine contribution to the communities where they live, work and play, regardless of the labels, diagnoses and prejudices which have excluded them in the past. This deceptively simple objective is, of course, remarkably difficult to achieve and implies the undoing of many decades of social policy whilst challenging deeply held prejudices and well-established structural and cultural discrimination in order to make genuine shifts in the service system. This is long-term committed work in which the person-centred plan is only a first step.

What then are the key characteristics of person-centred planning? First and foremost, person-centred planning is designed to promote inclusive lives for everyone: 'All means all!' In their work with disadvantaged school leavers, Beth Mount and Connie Lyle O'Brien (2002) talk about promoting five valued experiences:

1. Sharing places – sharing the ordinary places of community life at the same time and in the same way as others.

2. Belonging – developing a wide, diverse range of relationships with people with and without disabilities.

3. Being somebody – being respected by others and seen as a valued person who has positive roles to play in your life.

4. Choosing – making choices, big and small, in all areas of your life.

5. Contributing – contributing your gifts, talents, passions, interests, ideas and opinions to others in the community.

Second, person-centred planning is designed explicitly to help people make changes in their lives. It is not the function of person-centred planning to assess people or their service requirements. The key to achieving these aims is sometimes described as 'asking a different set of questions', questions grounded in:

- an imaginative and determined effort to discover a vision of a compelling future, which gives the person and their supporters something genuinely worth working towards

- a resolute focus on what the person has to offer. What are their strengths and gifts and where might these make a contribution to the wider community?

- the assumption that communities need diverse contributions

- finding and agreeing concrete first steps which the person can take with the practical and moral support of friends and allies.

Person-centred planning usually includes a meeting where these questions can be worked on with the person and their supporters. Two people who have a degree of independence should facilitate the meeting. One facilitator guides the process of the meeting, ensuring the person is genuinely at its heart and that people stick to the task. The other records the meeting on large pieces of wallpaper using words, symbols and pictures to create a live and memorable account of what has been discussed. The facilitators are guardians of the process and should challenge any tendency in the meeting to drift towards service-led solutions or away from the person's agenda. Effective plans are focused on real life, 'ordinary' goals such as fun and friends, work and achievement, moving house or going on holiday – the kinds of experiences we all value.

There are a number of different person-centred planning tools. They all share principles which are based on the values of inclusion and a commitment to help people achieve positive change in their lives. Those in commonest use in the UK at the present time are MAPs, PATH and Essential Lifestyles Planning. It is beyond the scope of this chapter to describe in detail how these approaches vary but their differences tend to reflect their origins and the context in which they were designed (for more on person-centred planning tools see Sanderson *et al.* 1997).

Each of the tools has strengths and weaknesses but in truth they share the same problems as paintbrushes and chisels; in some hands they create art and can empower and uplift, in others they can leave dispiriting damage. Facilitators may be skilful, knowledgeable and technically proficient and the resulting plans can look great, but if they do not hold to the values of inclusion for all, the 'product' can be a hollow shell. This is especially relevant to the present discussion. Where person-centred planning is implemented *for* or done *to* people, rather than *with* them, the outcomes will be less effective from their perspective, the only one which truly matters.

Person-centred planning and co-production
Genuinely with

Person-centred planning is at its most effective when it acts as a catalyst, promoting genuine partnership between professionals and the people they are trying to help. One way of understanding this process is as co-production in action. Lyle O'Brien and O'Brien (2002) comment that person-centred planning was intentionally designed to encourage human service workers to be more 'human' in their relationships to the people they serve. Recent feedback on work undertaken with young school leavers in Edinburgh (Weston 2005) included the following comments from young people:

> You spoke to me with respect and politeness and made me feel important.

> They treated us like adults.

The different questions which person-centred planning asks – about people's gifts and dreams, their passions and concerns, their story – shape this process. Instead of seeing clients, patients, consumers, service users and problem parents, we begin to see real people and therefore genuine potential partners. Person-centred planning is rooted in really careful listening, respect in all its complexity, and empathy for our fellow men and women. Kendrick (2000, p.4) describes this as 'personcenteredness': 'This quality could be thought of as the optimal or desirable ethical and values base of the kinds of people who tend to bring about improved respect and treatment for individuals. In this sense "personcenteredness" is a characteristic of people not systems.'

Sincere and thoughtful practitioners of person-centred planning invest time and energy genuinely working alongside people to build partnership. Helping the person prepare for the meeting might be about who they want to come, where they want the meeting and so on, but the person may also need time to work on their dream or think about what really makes sense to them. Facilitators do what it takes to give the person as much control and influence over the process as possible. When practitioners engage with people in this way and around the agenda created by these different questions, the relationship begins to shift subtly and become less like professional and client and more like genuine partners.

Case study 1

William was supported by a paid carer who lived near to his top floor tenement flat. This person helped him with a lot of practical everyday things but in many respects William was a very independent man who got around town a lot.

During our first planning meeting William was asked by others present about some of his preferences but he would invariably turn to me as the facilitator as though to ask, 'What do you think?' I would look back at him, all encouragement, and say with absolute sincerity, 'It's your meeting!' William would then grin knowingly and say with a shrug of the shoulders and heavy irony, 'Aye, so you say!'

I guess that, after 70 years of being told what to do and having people make decisions for him, it was going to take more than one person-centred planning meeting to convince William that we genuinely wanted him to be in charge.

We met six months after the first meeting to see how William was getting on. When we met to plan the second meeting, he showed me a small cupboard and the beautiful bone china tea set that was in immaculate condition in there. William smiled and said that he wanted to use this to make everyone a cup of tea when they came for his meeting the next week. It had been his mother's and my guess was that it had not seen a tealeaf since her death a few years earlier.

When I arrived for the meeting I was horrified that his carer had insisted on him putting it away in case he broke it. A swift debate followed during which I promised to help him with the teas and, in the end, William used his mother's best china for the refreshments at his meeting. He seemed pleased. My understanding of what had happened was that his decision to use the tea set was the beginnings of him believing it *was* his meeting.

Something worth working for

In order to make positive changes you need to have something worth working for. It is remarkable how often service interventions founder because they lack a clear and compelling vision. Do people get really excited about 'more respite' or 'increased one-to-one provision'? Most often, people are motivated by real life, meaningful goals like work, friends and foreign holidays. This is why person-centred planning approaches focus on dreams and aspirations.

Asking people about their dreams is much more than asking the person for a 'wish list'. It is about helping the person and their allies develop a sense of direction for the changes they want to make. All successful businesses work to a 'vision' – why shouldn't people who want to change their life for the better? If the person's dream seems far-distant or even fantastical, the job of those facilitating the plan is to help tease out the 'seeds' or 'threads' of that dream, so that these important elements can inform practical action planning.

> We asked Philip about his dream of being an actor; what do you really like about it? He wasn't bothered about being a celebrity. He wanted to get a message across to people – a message about equality and justice.

It is also very common for people's dreams to actually be very ordinary; what most of us would take for granted in our own lives.

> Tracey was really excited about leaving school and very clear about what she wanted to do, 'I want to work at Asda on the checkout!'

Some people fear that helping people to unfold their dreams might be harmful. From a family member's point of view, this is understandable because there may have been any number of dreams already squashed or discarded in a person's life. When such fears are present, it can be helpful to talk about these nightmares before thinking about the dream. Professionals who express similar concerns may be worried that they will be required to make dreams come true, when they already feel overloaded. Sometimes staff say that it is unfair to 'raise people's expectations' – again, perhaps, out of fear of the implications for their own role.

An undeniable consequence of effective person-centred planning is that people will change their expectations of what is good enough and begin to demand that services and staff respond better to what they want and need. This is a challenge which many staff will embrace and rise to – but for some it will be difficult and unwelcome. Empirical evidence shows that people with higher expectations, even apparently 'unrealistic' ones, will be more 'self-efficacious'. Bandura (1997) writes: 'A resilient sense of efficacy requires experience in overcoming obstacles through perseverant effort' (quoted in Lyte O'Brien and O'Brien 2002, p.281). Lowering expectations, as well-meaning professionals often do, is not only ethically questionable. It also actively undermines people's abilities to cope with further challenges in their lives.

Another factor which affects an individual's sense of empowerment and self-efficacy is how far the ambitions of the plan start to happen.

> Soon after his planning meeting Philip had the chance to appear as an extra in a TV show, but he wants to keep his options open. He has begun studying art at a local FE College and has also led workshops at two national conferences and given presentations about person-centred planning to young people and families. His dreams have yet to come true in a literal sense, but there can be little doubt that they have shaped and influenced the manner in which he has grasped the opportunities that have come his way.

Some people – whether or not they have a label of disability – may need a lot of help to think in this way. Some of us are great dreamers (how interesting that such an observation can have negative connotations in our culture) whilst others find it harder. Some people's dreams lie buried deep and negative life experiences make this more likely.

Creating a vision is at the heart of person-centred planning, and is also a particularly effective way of engaging with people in a co-productive manner.

Focus on strengths not deficiencies

Traditional professional cultures and ways of engagement relentlessly focus on people's deficiencies not their strengths. This is partly dictated by circumstances; if people did not need some kind of support to do things they would presumably get on and do them. However, the deficiency-led assessment is so deeply entrenched in policies, procedures and resource-allocating models in health and social care that it can both diminish the humanity of its 'clients' and undermine their ability to make a contribution both to their own welfare and to the wider community. Often families and individuals feel 'assessed to death', yet discover that this leads to no practical help at all or to the allocation of a service which at best approximates the help required. This can be profoundly disempowering.

Person-centred planning focuses immediately on the half-full portion of the glass. What does this person have to offer? Pearpoint and Snow (1998) comment:

> Everyone has gifts – countless ordinary and extraordinary gifts. A gift is anything that one is, or has, or does that creates an opportunity for a meaningful interaction with at least one other person. There are two gifts that ALL

people have and that every other gift depends on. The first is presence. Since you are here, you are embodying the possibility of a meaningful interaction with someone else. Secondly, you are different from everyone else – in countless ways. Difference is required to make meaning possible. This means that human interaction arises from presence and difference. (p.167)

Focusing on the person's strengths, passions, interests and the things that others like and admire about them provides a tremendous starting point for a co-productive relationship.

During Philip's plan, one of his teachers added, 'He does fly off the handle a bit sometimes.' The facilitator asked where this would be a gift. 'Well, he really hates to see folk being treated unfairly or picked on…', at which point Philip added, 'I hate bullies!' By this stage many present were nodding agreement. His teacher summed up, 'Yeah, he rages against injustice!' That sounded a lot better – it was also more accurate.

The other linked assumption in person-centred planning is that communities are predisposed to invite or welcome contribution.

Lucy and her family returned with a beautiful abstract painting she had done. The other members of the group were really impressed with her work. Lucy's mum said that she wanted to have it framed and donate it to the nearby home for older people. Some of those present suggested finding a gallery to show and possibly sell the painting. Options seemed to increase with every suggestion someone made.

Team work

Person-centred planning is a way of building a team around a person to help them make the changes they want in their lives. Mount and Lyle O'Brien (2002) describe this as an *intervisionary* rather than a *multi-disciplinary* team. A diverse group which can think in terms of ordinary solutions and can contribute to action planning works best in person-centred planning. Comments from the evaluation of a planning project with young people illustrate the value of teamwork:

Everyone was in one room; everyone heard what Nicola's worries were.

The plan was opening up avenues; people will do something to help him. People were saying…we're willing to help with this and that…they were going out of their way.

In recent planning with young people and their families, the presence of involved professionals, whilst helpful, was by no means essential to the effective working of the group. However, the presence of close family, siblings and a friend or two has been invaluable.

When people's planning meetings are dominated by professionals, the outcomes are less effective. Workers can jump to service solutions, for example a person talks about making friends and a befriender is suggested. When most of the action points are delegated to people in their professional roles, the meeting takes on the semblance of a traditional review, with less likelihood that actions will be followed through. These problems can arise because the other people in the person's life have not been invited to contribute. If the person is isolated from family and community and has no one else in their 'team', supporting professionals need to develop long-term strategies to broaden the person's connectedness.

The added bonus of person-centred planning is its invitation to families, communities and people themselves to join in the decision making and action planning processes. Often, family, friends and professionals are surprised how people, when invited to take centre stage, grasp the opportunity with open arms. This approach of inviting contribution, developing teamwork and encouraging peer support is not unique to person-centred planning. For example, Family Group Conferencing was first developed in New Zealand and is now practised internationally. It starts from an assumption that young people and their families and networks will have inherent strengths that can be overlooked or bypassed by services intent on 'sorting' young people who are in danger of falling into the youth justice system. Ten years after the legislation mandating the Family Group Conferencing approach, Mike Doolan, a former Chief Social Worker in New Zealand, says that: 'The capacity of families to take control continues to astound us; families can make safe decisions for young people and are experts about themselves' (1999).

Some approaches to person-centred planning consciously encourage peer support by bringing several teams together over a number of sessions to work through the stages of the planning process. In their analysis of a decade of this work in New York, Lyle O'Brien and O'Brien (2002, pp.282–3) draw on Bandura (1997) to describe the four kinds of experience which these sessions support.

1. Over the five months of the programme participants can acquire skills, abilities and strengths to overcome obstacles and difficulties through sustained effort. Bandura calls these *mastery experiences.*

2. Seeing other young people and parents in similar situations succeed through perseverance, models skills and strategies which other participants can learn. Bandura calls this *vicarious experience.*

3. Having opportunities in a relatively safe environment to have successes which are acknowledged by others who can confirm their confidence in participants' abilities to manage changing situations. Bandura calls this *social persuasion.*

4. Having opportunities in the group to learn that physical and emotional reactions to difficult situations can be a source of positive energy for action rather than reasons to despair or give up. Bandura talks about this as *physiological and emotional states.*

Our experience of similar processes in the UK (for more see Coulson and Simmons 2006) echoes the American evaluations. One participant in the first group in Redcar and Cleveland summed up the impact of participation as 'hope, optimism and imagination'.

Problems in practice

Glancing at recent social work and disability publications, you could be forgiven for thinking that person-centred planning was 'the next big thing'. It was not always so. In the past decade, person-centred planning has moved from the radical fringes of human services, where it was often ignored, dismissed as 'unrealistic', or at best seen as something a bit American and exotic, to become extremely fashionable. By 2001 the *Valuing People* report (Department of Health 2001) lent explicit endorsement to person-centred planning. The *Same as You* report in Scotland (Scottish Executive 2000) was less specific but clearly endorsed a move towards individuals having a more active role in planning their own lives.

In the period before this high-level endorsement, thousands of service professionals in social work, health and education (and smaller numbers of family members) had been introduced to the ideas of person-centred planning through the efforts of pioneering UK organisations and regular visits to Britain of leading practitioners from the USA and Canada. In 2005 the Institute for Health Research (IHR) published a report on the impact of person-centred planning which concludes:

> Very little change was apparent in people's lives prior to the introduction of person centred planning. After the introduction of person centred planning, significant positive changes were found in the areas of: social networks; contact with family; contact with friends; community based activities; scheduled day activities; and levels of choice. (Elliott *et al.* 2005)

Nevertheless, at the very moment person-centred planning appears to have become the accepted, commonsense approach, the values which underpin it are in danger of dilution. Organisational commitment to person-centred planning is seldom utterly cynical, but the ideas can be applied in ways which make success unlikely and which foster cynicism about the approach and – more worryingly – about the goal of inclusion. The IHR report cautions that 'Person centred planning may be helpful but is not sufficient condition to promote social inclusion.'

When a good idea is embraced by large bureaucracies, it has a tendency to distort to fit the system which has adopted it. While there is evidence of the person-centred approach contributing to systemic change, there is also considerable evidence of person-centred planning being assimilated by the system in ways which undermine the intentions of its champions.

Somehow, the message that everyone should have access to person-centred planning morphs into: everyone will have a person-centred plan whether they want one or not! This derives from a tick-box approach to measuring outcomes which agencies develop or have to comply with; that is, we are doing a great job because 99.5 per cent of our residents have got a plan. Of course the point is what percentage have a life! As Smull (2002, p.59) says in the title of his article, 'A plan is not an outcome!'

Large agencies invest a great deal of energy in working out where person-centred planning fits with existing frameworks for assessment and planning. For example, when the notion of Single Shared Assessment was introduced by the Scottish Executive, some local areas attempted to graft aspects of person-centred planning on to this model. The result resembles the galaxy-devouring Borg in *Star Trek* who assimilate all life-forms in their own image. Person-centred planning does not neatly fit with Single Shared Assessment because it is not assessment. It is more than incongruous to ask someone what they are really passionate or interested in, then go on to ask them what their bathing or toileting needs are.

Agencies also 'codify' the approach to planning, by developing packs, guidelines, frameworks, pro-formas etc. The intention to achieve clarity and consistency when delivering a service to people is good. However, the result can be people following the rules in a formulaic way. This is a long way from a constellation of tools.

As person-centred planning has become more popular it becomes more difficult for professionals to admit to a lack of expertise in this new technique. The desire to 'acquire' person-centred planning for a professional CV encourages a focus on technical skills and procedures, rather than on the spirit of enquiry, humility and partnership. Service workers rapidly appropriate the surface trappings of person-centred planning, before they have wrestled with the major implications of person-centredness for their job and services in which they work.

However, the most fundamental factor in undermining the impact of person-centred planning is the lack of responsiveness of human service and other service systems to the kinds of lives people want. Nothing undermines the efficacy of a person-centred approach more; families and individuals are encouraged to have the courage to say what they want, often after years of feeling ignored, only to find barriers in the way of what they want to achieve, which are usually summarised in three words: lack of resources. Whilst this phrase is sometimes only too true it can also be used as an excuse to do nothing. People should not embark on person-centred planning without commitment from those around the person to do everything they can to make some change in the positive direction the person identifies.

Conclusion

In the past few years person-centred planning has become increasingly 'fashionable' in human services. This is to be welcomed, but person-centred planning is no more than a good idea and like others can be distorted when large bureaucratic systems try to make them their own. Its aims might be undermined by its co-option into the very system it really ought to challenge and change in order to enable people to have better lives.

In arguing for the art and soul of this work, people like John O'Brien, Connie Lyle O'Brien and Beth Mount are trying to defend this groundbreaking work from becoming little more than a (big) paper exercise. We need to be creative and artful if we genuinely want to work with people in sincere partnership. If we find ways to do this well and people are genuinely engaged in the co-production of their own welfare our services and society may take a significant shift towards becoming person centred in more than just words.

References

Bandura, A. (1997) *Self-Efficacy: The Exercise of Control*. New York, NY: Worth Publishers.

Coulson, S. and Simmons, H. (2006) *The Big Plan – A Good Life after School*. Toronto: Inclusion Press.

Department of Health (2001) *Valuing People: A New Strategy for Learning Disability for the 21st Century*. London: Department of Health.

Doolan, M. (1999) 'The Family Group Conference – 10 years on.' www.restorative.org, accessed on 7 September 2007.

Elliott, J., Emerson, E., Robertson, J., Hatton, C. *et al.* (2005) *The Impact of Person Centred Planning*. Lancaster: Institute for Health Research.

Falvey, M.A., Forest, M., Pearpoint, J. and Rosenberg, R.L. (2003) *All My Life's a Circle – Using the Tools: MAPS & PATHS*. Toronto: Inclusion Press.

Kendrick, M. (2000) *When People Matter More Than Systems*. Keynote presentation for 'The Promise of Opportunity' Conference, 27–28 March, Albany, NY.

Lyle O'Brien, C. and O'Brien, J. (2002) 'Large Group Process for Person-Centered Planning.' In J. O'Brien and C. Lyle O'Brien (eds) *Implementing Person-Centered Planning: The Voices of Experience*. Toronto: Inclusion Press.

McKnight, J. (1995) *The Careless Society: Community and its Counterfeits*. New York, NY: Basic Books.

Mount, B. and Lyle O'Brien, C. (2002) *Building New Worlds*. Amenia, NY: Capacity Works.

Pearpoint, J. and Snow, J. (1998) *From Behind the Piano. And What's Really Worth Doing and How to Do It*. Toronto: Inclusion Press.

Sanderson, H., Kennedy, J., Ritchie, P. and Goodwin, G. (1997) *People, Plans and Possibilities*. Edinburgh: Scottish Human Services.

Scottish Executive (2000) *The Same as You? A Review of Services for People with Learning Disabilities*. Edinburgh: Scottish Executive.

Smull, M. (2002) 'A Plan Is Not an Outcome.' In J. O'Brien and C. Lyle O'Brien (eds) *Implementing Person-Centered Planning: The Voices of Experience*. Toronto: Inclusion Press.

Weston, J. (2005) *Future Plans Evaluation*. Edinburgh: Edinburgh Development Group.

CHAPTER 8

Restoring 'Stakeholder' Involvement in Justice

Bill Whyte

Introduction

Crime is a major focus of political and public concern at the beginning of the twenty-first century in the UK and is a prime area of public anxiety. Youth crime and anti-social behaviour, in particular, have become a key focus for politicians keen to demonstrate to potential voters that they have the policy and service solutions to community problems (Scottish Executive 2006, p.23). The predominance of 'punishment' as a cultural response in the UK to criminal behaviour has meant that often the public framing of provision for responding to crime has been dominated by retributive justice principles without consideration on how best to respond effectively to the characteristics and circumstances of those involved. Adversarial criminal justice often attracts the general criticism that it provides limited opportunity for 'user' or 'stakeholder' involvement in decision making and that retributive criminal processes tend to exclude those with the greatest stake, the victim and other interested parties, and limits the opportunity for communities of interest to resolve their own social problems. Developments in community justice in western jurisdictions, for example neighbourhood courts, various forms of volunteer decision-making panels and even peer courts, reflect this dissatisfaction with formal criminal justice processes and are attempting to give communities a greater stake in their own social well-being and community safety.

The goal of community justice initiatives is to empower citizens, voluntary groups and neighbourhood associations as partners in the justice process. They tend to be organised around principles of 'localism', with the focus on neighbourhood initiatives to create more accessible and less formal provision aimed at shifting decisions to the locality affected directly by the crime. The growth and development of a more distinctive 'lay' involvement in decision making in justice arenas is often aimed at preventing prosecution, at decriminalisation, and at reducing the associated negative amplification effects of criminal processes for people who offend, particularly young people. However, the term 'community member' in such initiatives is generally confined to people who have no direct personal involvement in the crime even though they may represent the community in some sense.

Developments in restorative practices in justice, such as victim mediation and restorative conferencing, are geared to involve adults or young people who have offended with parents, families, victims and community members directly involved with or affected by the crime. These 'stakeholders' or 'communities of interest' are placed, as far as possible, at the heart of the decision-making process on the assumption that this is likely to be a more effective way of problem resolution, leading to greater satisfaction with the process and resulting in some healing and enhancement of social integration and community cohesion. This emphasis on involving those most affected by crime has resulted in an increased use of restorative practices by justice systems, schools and community groups and has provided a focus for a debate about who should 'own' and take responsibility for social conflict and crime and about the boundaries and potential of restorative practices, however defined.

> The purpose of this shift is the return of ownership of crime problems and their solutions to those individuals and groups who are most affected by the behaviours at hand, and who have the most at stake in finding a satisfactory solution. (LaPrairie 1998, p.65)

Greater emphasis on partnership between communities and the justice system can be seen as a search for mutual and collaborative advantage between the state and communities of interest. This is a recognition, implicitly or explicitly, that while the state has a major role in creating conditions for promoting social well-being and community safety, communities of interest must be co-producers in decision making and responses if more effective and lasting solutions to local crime-related problems are to be found. In this way restorative practices rely on co-production to achieve a dynamic process and mutually beneficial outcomes for participants that state processes cannot achieve on their own. Restorative practices in youth crime are consistent with the UN

Convention on the Rights of the Child (1989) and the international standards set by the UN regulations which encourage the use of extra-judicial solutions and socio-educational approaches to mobilise family and community resources in assisting resolution and better integration of those involved in crime.

The remainder of this chapter examines restorative practices as a form of co-production and the extent to which they can provide better direction in justice and collaborative advantage, influenced by principles of resolution, healing and integration of all parties, particularly the people who offend and are victims.[1]

Restorative practices

Restorative justice is a response to crime that considers the needs of victims, those who offend and the community (Zehr 2002). It is an attempt to put into practice a set of ethical ideas about how human beings should relate to each other and, in particular, to those who present trouble, seeking to resolve and strengthen relationships where possible. Restorative practices are designed to give victims of crime an opportunity to tell the offender about the impact of their actions on them and their families, and to encourage acceptance of responsibility for, and to repair, the harm they have caused. Its general aims are to 'address' the harm done, to restore, to varying degrees, the relationship between the persons harmed and harming that was disturbed by the offence, to reduce re-offending and to improve their experience of the criminal justice system (Marshall 1999).

The term 'restorative practice' is used to refer to a diverse range of formal and informal practices, all of which, in their purist form, rely on the combined efforts of participants to co-produce shared understanding and mutually beneficial outcomes that could not be achieved by more formal and traditional state processes. These include:

- victim/offender mediation (VOM), restorative and family conferences in criminal and youth justice

- truth and reconciliation processes and peace movements in South Africa and Northern Ireland

---

1   The terms 'victim' and 'offender' are used hereafter for simplicity; this risks narrowly labelling them when it is their range of qualities and characteristics that are crucial to co-production in restorative practice.

- community mediation and discretionary problem solving including policing initiatives in disputes between citizens
- restorative practices for children in trouble at school.

There is a plethora of descriptors for the varying practices that claim to fall within the ambit of restorative practices within adult or youth justice, including mediation and reparation, family group conferencing, restorative and community conferencing, restorative cautions, sentencing and healing circles, community panels or courts, and other communitarian associations (Braithwaite 1999). While restorative practices often provide alternatives to formal justice processes, in some jurisdictions they are police-led, for example Thames Valley restorative cautioning, and in others are incorporated within formal justice processes with explicit justice objectives including punishment and retribution as part of formal judicial disposals (Daly and Hayes 2001).

Victim–offender mediation (VOM) provides a range of options aimed at including victims in the justice process as central to the approach. At one end of the range VOM may simply involve the offender writing a letter of apology to his or her victim. At the other end, it can involve a structured meeting or conference between the victim, offender and other interested parties, in which the impact of the offence is examined more closely by all concerned.

Family group conferences (FGC) are generally modelled on an approach developed in New Zealand and bring together family members of both the offender, victim, friends, people from the local community, and professional social workers or justice personnel to look at the facts: what happened and why; the consequences: how the victim and others were affected; and the future: how the person can make amends, in an effort to produce a mutually satisfactory resolution.

Restorative justice conferences (RJC) are intended to enable victims, offender and their respective families or support people to actively participate in the process of addressing the harm caused by the offence, to talk about why an event occurred and how it affected them, and to decide on a plan of action, which may specify what needs to be done to put right the harm and to prevent it happening in the future. The agreed plan should, as far as possible, be based on a consensus of views of those at the meeting and will usually outline what is to happen and who is to oversee or support those taking action to ensure that the plan is carried out. The plan may include compensating the victim, family and/or friends changing their routines to provide support and encouragement to both victim and offender, the provision of practical and financial assistance or other services by statutory authorities or other agencies and involvement in local programmes. In some jurisdictions the plan is presented to professionals or to a court who will normally accept it as part of the final disposal.

These types of restorative practices place a very clear focus on the co-production of mutually beneficial outcomes through direct participation of the people most affected by the event and on personal 'uplift' achieved in taking responsibility for problem resolution while supported and affirmed by families or other positive social supports. It is not always possible, however, to involve victims or other supporters directly in restorative practices and a level of co-production is sought through variations of this approach. In the case of damage to community property, for example, a representative such as a teacher from the school involved may attend and represent the victim perspective. In some circumstances, victims and the person meet without support persons. In this case 'face-to-face' meetings are made available supported by trained staff. Shuttle mediation provides another model where the offender does not come face to face with their victim but someone, usually a trained person, 'shuttles' information between the two key participants to achieve a satisfactory outcome.

Police-led conferencing was developed in Wagga Wagga, New South Wales, in 1991 as part of police cautioning. This type of approach has no explicit aim of repairing family or social bonds and often follows a 'script' directing the order and form of communication in a safe and constructive way. Restorative warnings in youth justice are formal police cautions that attempt to engage in a structured discussion with the young person and their family about the harm caused by the offence, its consequences for victims and how the harm might be repaired. Victims are seldom involved directly. This approach has been pioneered in a number of areas in England, most notably by Thames Valley Police, and it is now a key element of the work of the Youth Justice Board throughout England and Wales (Hoyle and Young 2002). From 2004 all police warnings for young people in Scotland adopted restorative methods, drawing on the experience of Thames Valley Police. While it could be argued that such processes really do not conform to requirements of restorative practice as a form of co-production, they nonetheless attempt to promote and support new understanding and change through the dynamic generated by the process.

Rationale: Restorative values and principles

Restorative practices in justice operate on the premise that crime and conflict creates harm for individuals and communities and fractures social relationships. It seeks to balance the concerns of the victim and the community with the need to better integrate the offender within a community or society. If conflict is viewed as an opportunity for individuals and communities to learn to take individual or shared responsibility for the harm done, then an important outcome for any effective process or approach should be to assist those involved to grow and to have their needs addressed. Similarly it can be argued that, with children and young people, it is in their best interests to understand the harm done and its consequences on self and others as an important element in social and moral development and to have the positive opportunity to share in the resolution of the harm with the support of family or significant others as a way of building personal and social 'capital' and a sense of personal efficacy.

These outcomes are best achieved through forms of co-production in which the needs of all those affected by the harm should be central and commentators on restorative practice emphasise the importance of placing key stakeholders at the forefront of the process and shaping of the resolution.

> Restorative justice is a process to involve, to the extent possible, those who have a stake in a specific offence and to collectively identify and address harms, needs, and obligations, in order to heal and put things as right as possible. (Zehr 2002, p.37)

In this sense restorative practices are intended to be holistic, addressing the repercussions and obligations created by harm directly. When compared with retributive justice models, restorative approaches seek to achieve a paradigm shift in thinking about effective responses to harm. This becomes most apparent when comparing the values and principles of restorative practices to those of the criminal or youth justice systems:

> Restorative justice is fundamentally different from retributive justice. It is justice that puts energy into the future, not into what is past. It focuses on what needs to be healed, what needs to be repaid, what needs to be learned in the wake of crime. It looks at what needs to be strengthened if such things are not to happen again. (Sharpe 1998, p.7)

Such comments serve to re-emphasise the view that formal justice practices often create dissatisfaction by detaching the interest of stakeholders, victims, offender and others from decision making and the outcome, or from any concern that stakeholders might in some ways be better off or 'improved' by the process.

Restorative justice has been promoted as a more 'culturally sensitive' model of justice, particularly for ethnic groups and socially marginalised people who are over-represented in criminal justice in most jurisdictions, and one which can serve communities more effectively than a justice system that seems to discriminate rather than integrate. While the modern restorative justice movement began in the 1970s, it can be argued that restorative practice has been a dominant model of justice throughout most of human history, for perhaps all of the world's peoples; one that has been lost in modern society (Braithwaite 2002; Zehr 2002). For example, traditional Maori practice involved victims, offenders and families of both, first in acknowledging guilt and expressing remorse and, second, in finding ways to restore the social balance so that the victim could be compensated by the group and the offender reintegrated within the social group (Maxwell and Morris 1993). In Scotland the judicial practice of assythment, only formally abolished in 1976, allowed victims of crime and their relatives, in certain circumstances, to claim financial or material remedy from perpetrators. This was an ancient mechanism whereby wrongs from murder to causal injury could be dealt with by negotiation with the relevant parties with or without Crown or state intervention. It provided an acceptable means of avoiding a blood feud, since becoming a victim of crime could be the consequence of kinship activities or of being a member of a collective entity or clan (McKay 1992, p.242).

While it is important not to romanticise or overstretch the meaning of these ancient methods, they seem, symbolically at least, concerned with the restoration of community cohesion and community well-being – in modern language a safer, better society – as much as for individual restoration. Their reliance on mutually agreed and co-produced outcomes has the potential to reinforce integrative social values in the best interest of the community that formal retributive approaches, which often threaten everyone and removes the 'community of interest' from the process, in many circumstances fail to achieve. Zehr (2001) has argued that the failure in criminal justice has resulted in a crisis of an old paradigm requiring radical change.

What is restorative? Theoretical directions

The discussion above begs the question: when is a practice in justice restorative? There is no universally accepted or concise definition and practices vary greatly in their apparent intention. Marshall's definition appears to encompass the main generally accepted principles of restorative justice:

> Restorative justice is a process whereby all the parties with a stake in a particular offence come together to resolve collectively how to deal with the aftermath of the offence and its implications for the future. (Cited in Braithwaite 1999, p.5)

The United Nations *Draft Declaration on Basic Principles on the Use of Restorative Justice Programmes in Criminal Matters* (1999) defines restorative justice as a process in which the victim, offender and/or any other individuals or community members affected by a crime participate actively together in the resolution of matters arising from the crime, often with the help of a fair and impartial third party.

While collaboration and co-production are central concepts, neither of these definitions stresses social or community cohesion as an essential characteristic of restorative practice and the UN definition places little emphasis on mutually beneficial outcomes. It could be argued to be important if restorative practices are to be more than simply a satisfactory or humanising practice within a retributive justice system and actually offer a new paradigm for justice rather than simply an attempt to salvage the existing paradigm by providing more meaningful practices alongside punishment and retribution. For many it is precisely the traditional criminal justice agencies which need to be disengaged and changed if the victim, offender and the community of interest are to recapture ownership for resolving the conflict (Wright 1999).

Restorative practices are not the practical or applied outgrowth of any particular criminological or criminal justice theory but have emerged from a variety of sources through a shared frustration with criminal justice and through seeking practical ways of having a positive impact on people. Marshall draws attention to the pluralistic nature of the many restorative justice initiatives currently being practised in the UK, Australasia and North America.

> Restorative justice is not, therefore, a single academic theory of crime or justice, but represents, in a more or less eclectic way, the accretion of actual experience in working successfully with particular crime problems. (1999, p.7)

Nonetheless, for many advocates, for justice to be restorative it must evidence the consistent involvement of all parties affected by the crime, and focus on the development, implementation and maintenance of mutual healing, reparation and satisfaction rather than retribution and punishment (Schiff 1998). There have to be benefits or 'uplift' at least for the two main characters: the person who causes harm and the person who experiences it. This mutuality needs to be maintained in any balanced system of restorative justice and is not necessarily present in many practices incorporated into formal criminal legal processes (Bazemore and Umbreit 1994).

Braithwaite's (1989) theory of 're-integrative shaming' argues that people are generally not deterred from committing crime by the threat of official punishment but by the two informal processes of social control: fear of social disapproval and social conscience. Through restorative practice the offender is made powerfully aware of the disapproval of their actions by significant others in their lives. The potentially alienating and stigmatising effects of shaming are overcome by re-acceptance and affirmation of the person's value in the social community. Agreements reached by family members, friends or other individuals important to the offender are likely to be more effective and lasting in their impact than those imposed by an impersonal legal institution. For most people, he argues, the fear of being shamed by those they care about may be a major deterrent to committing crime because the opinions of family and friends mean more than those of an unknown criminal justice authority. By including supporters, restorative conferences allow people to be held responsible in the context of a community of care as well of concern. This is essentially co-produced and cannot simply be required or imposed.

Gottfredson and Hirschi (1990) argue that the key factor distinguishing those who obey the law from those who break it is self-control. As they see it, self-control begins to be learned during the early years of childhood in the course of social interaction. Most people develop sufficient self-control to live sociably. Those relatively few people who fail to develop adequate self-control tend 'to avoid attachment to or involvement in all social institutions' (1990, p.168). The resulting 'tendency of people most in need of the restraining influence of family, school and friendship to be outside of those spheres of influence is a matter of considerable importance' (ibid.). Not only do restorative practices provide an opportunity for people to accept their share of responsibility for their actions, it also affords them the opportunity, where possible, to repair the harm they have caused with the support of their families while involving victims in the process, strengthening their sense of social cohesion, self-efficacy and responsibility. Informal and restorative practice generally seeks social involvement and social integration providing a psycho-social means to distinguish that which is socially appropriate from that which is not. From these perspectives, in contrast, formal, official punishment seeks public shaming and to stigmatise those who have transgressed the law. It aims to separate and distinguish them from the law-abiding majority. It does this in varying degrees, all of which are degrading. The more severe forms of public shaming and stig-matisation involve temporary removal and exclusion from society through deprivation of liberty in the form of imprisonment.

If restorative practice is to offer a new paradigm to modify the foundations of the criminal justice system and fulfil the requirements to make victim and offender better after the process by repairing harm, making amends, promoting prevention and desistence, what place does punishment have? Some commenta-tors argue that restorative practice in justice can be just another kind of punishment and that reparation can convey 'pay back time' much in the way of traditional retributive attitudes.

While most advocates of restorative practice reject punishment and infliction of pain as an objective, there is recognition that true empathy with the person harmed and feelings of remorse will be painful. For this reason restorative responses should be proportionate in their demand and expectation. Daly (2003) argues that restorative practice within state mechanisms is intended to be a punishment, albeit an alternative punishment that is not humiliating, harming or degrading and that it should combine retribution and rehabilitation. Commentators like Duff (1996) have sought to reconcile these kinds of positions by arguing that, while true repentance cannot be coerced, punishment including the infliction of pain is communicative and encourages repentance and forgiveness which are conducive to possible reconciliation and repairing harm, which ideally the offender imposes on himself. Strong psychological evidence can be cited to challenge such a view and to argue that punishment does not deter the most recalcitrant but simply gives the 'ordinary' person good reason for compliance (Andrews and Bonta 2003). Punishment in a counter-productive way tends to induce resistance, resentment and strategies to avoid pain not necessarily related to change objectives, and so inhibits learning rather than enhancing it.

Restorative outcomes

Braithwaite's review of the evidence reached encouraging, though cautious, conclusions about the efficacy of restorative justice (Braithwaite 1989). Only one of more than thirty studies he examined could be interpreted as showing an increase in re-offending for any type of offender involved in restorative practices and many showed reduced offending. While restitution appears an important motivator for victim participation, data suggest it is less important to victims than the opportunity to talk about the offence and its impact (Bazemore and Umbreit 2001).

The Canberra Re-Integrative Shaming Experiments (RISE) concluded that both offenders and victims found conferences to be procedurally fairer and more satisfactory than a court process (Sherman, Strang and Moore 2000). The study reported a substantial drop in offending rates by violent offenders (by 38 crimes per 100 per year) relative to the effect of being sent to court. However, a small increase in re-offending was reported by drink drivers (by 6 crimes per 100 offenders per year). For juvenile property offences (shoplifting and personal offences) no differences in offending rates was found between court and conference groups on the basis of one-year before–after changes.

In a study in Glasgow (Dutton and Whyte 2006) involving 1236 young people aged 15 and under, who were first or minor offenders, of the 645 diverted to restorative police warnings, 73 per cent were not re-referred for offending in the subsequent 12-month period. Compared to the previous year when restorative options were not available, of 1695 young people diverted simply by a warning letter to parents, 68 per cent were not re-referred in the subsequent 12-month period. Consistently high levels of satisfaction with the restorative processes were recorded from police, young people and victims.

Aggregating data from a range of studies (meta-analysis) provides the most promising approach for establishing outcomes and controlling for key variables in restorative practices. Two reviews (Latimer, Dowden and Muise 2005; Rowe 2002) concluded that the young people involved in restorative practices acquired a greater understanding of the harm they had done, acquired feelings of empathy towards the people or organisations they harmed and were less likely to engage in future criminal behaviour. There is to date no research in the literature that examines the longer-term effects for victims who participate in restorative practices in justice.

Despite encouraging research findings, critics point to a variety of dangers and possible unintended outcomes both for offenders and for their victims (Minor and Morrison 1996; O'Connor 1997; Wundersitz 1997). There is the potential for victims to be 'revictimised' during conferences and emerge more traumatised or fearful than before, especially if they are faced by an unrepentant and belligerent respondent. Concerns have also been raised about legal rights under conferencing models, that young people in particular may end up receiving 'excessive punishment' at the hands of vengeful victims. Furthermore, the process can be dominated by professionals, resulting in questionable pressure, intentional or unintentional, placed on people to accept guilt for the offence. A lack of available welfare and family support services can result in more shaming and restitution than assistance and social integration.

Restorative practices have become fully embedded in legislation in youth justice practice in many jurisdictions such as New Zealand, England and Wales and Northern Ireland. Evaluation of 46 schemes funded by the Youth Justice Board in England and Wales found a tendency to rely too heavily on community reparation and a low level of direct involvement of victims in meeting with their offenders (Crawford and Newburn 2003). Research on the Thames Valley restorative police cautions found no better outcomes than for traditional cautioning and suggested that police practices may result in net widening when they represent simply an adaptation to existing justice practice rather than an alternative to prosecution (Wilcox, Young and Hoyle 2004). Similarly critics claim that restorative initiatives, particularly in the US, are too state driven and to that extent represent an extension of existing criminal justice approaches – new names for unchanged practice – rather than a new paradigm and approach to community justice (McCold 2004) where community initiatives simply transfer powers to community 'strangers'.

Conclusion

Restorative practices represent a form of co-production either as part of or as an alternative to mainstream or traditional justice practice and are generally considered an improvement on mainstream court-dominated systems. Restorative practice appears to open ways of dealing with the aftermath of crime that are more satisfactory for victims, more constructive for communities and society and more integrative for offenders. Those most affected by crime are at the heart of the process and are supported to be part of the solution by being involved in meaningful social interactions with the capacity to hold to account and to support reparative action.

Restorative practice means different things to different people but in most of its guises it presents challenges to establishment thinking on justice, particularly on how to achieve a constructive shift from sterile punishment to better forms of problem resolution and social integration. Restorative practices have the potential to provide a form of partnership between the state and individuals, families and communities as co-producers, whereby people can participate as citizens and stakeholders with expert knowledge and not simply as passive recipients of justice.

Studies in restorative practices are plagued with methodological difficulties which make firm conclusions impossible. Nonetheless, for individuals who choose to participate in restorative practices in justice, studies produce consistently encouraging results against four major objectives of victim satisfaction, offender satisfaction, restitution compliance and re-offending. A key ingredient seems to be direct victim–offender involvement. Taken as a whole, existing data on the impact of restorative practices in justice is positive in direction but uncertain and still subject to investigation, particularly in regard to young people involved in less serious offending.

While the effects of restorative practices on recidivism remain somewhat uncertain, proponents have consistently argued that it is naive to believe that a time-limited restorative intervention will have a dramatic effect on altering longstanding criminal and delinquent behaviour (Umbreit 1996). There is little evidence to date that restorative practices have had a major impact on sentencing or re-offending in the UK where prison populations remain extraordinarily high. Outcome data would suggest that, where intervention is necessary, restorative practices provide a positive methodology. However, because practices are restorative is not a justification or reason for intervention in itself.

A further attraction or limitation of restorative practice, depending on one's standpoint, is that it provides a 'world-view' across the political spectrum. On the one hand the greater role given to victims is supported by the so-called 'law-and-order lobby' and victim support groups concerned about perceived weak penalties from criminal courts. On the other hand groups such as youth advocacy and welfare are attracted to the diversionary uses of restorative practice. Anything that unites and is seen to meet the objectives of the political right and left in the UK, USA, Australia and New Zealand has to be treated with some caution and has to be subjected to critical evaluation in its implementation in any given social context.

References

Andrews, D.A. and Bonta, J. (2003) *The Psychology of Criminal Conduct* (3rd edn). Cincinnati, OH: Anderson.

Bazemore, G. and Umbreit, M. (1994) *Balanced and Restorative Justice.* Washington, DC: Department of Justice, Office of Justice Programs.

Bazemore, G. and Umbreit, M. (2001) *A Comparison of Four Restorative Conferencing Models.* Washington, DC: US Department of Justice.

Braithwaite, J. (1989) *Crime, Shame, and Reintegration.* Cambridge: Cambridge University Press.

Braithwaite, J. (1999) 'Restorative Justice: Assessing Optimistic and Pessimistic Accounts.' In M. Tonry (ed.) *Crime and Justice: A Review of Research.* Chicago, IL: University of Chicago Press.

Braithwaite, J. (2002) *Restorative Justice and Responsive Regulation.* New York, NY: Oxford University Press.

Crawford, A. and Newburn, T. (2003) *Youth Offending and Restorative Justice: Implementing Reform in Youth Justice.* London: Willan Publishing.

Daly, K. (2003) 'Restorative Justice: The Real Story.' In G. Johnstone (ed.) *A Restorative Justice Reader.* Cullompton: Willan Publishing.

Daly, K. and Hayes, H. (2001) 'Restorative Justice and Conferencing in Australia.' *Trends and Issues 186.* Canberra: Australian Institute of Criminology.

Duff, R.A. (1996) *Criminal Attempts.* Oxford: Clarendon Press.

Dutton, K. and Whyte, B. (2006) *Implementing Restorative Justice within an Integrated Welfare System: The Evaluation of Glasgow's Restorative Justice Service, Interim Summary Report.* Edinburgh: CJSWDC.

Gottfredson, M.R. and Hirschi, T. (1990) *A General Theory of Crime.* Stanford: Stanford University Press.

Hoyle, C. and Young, R. (2002) 'Restorative Justice: Assessing the Prospects and Pitfalls.' In M. McConville and G. Wilson (eds) *The Handbook of the Criminal Justice Process.* Oxford: Oxford University Press.

Latimer, J., Dowden, C. and Muise, D. (2005) *The Effectiveness of Restorative Justice Practices: A Meta-Analysis.* Ottawa, ON: Canadian Department of Justice.

LaPrairie, C. (1998) 'The new justice: some implications for Aboriginal communities.' *Canadian Journal of Criminology 40,* 1, 61–79.

Marshall, T. (1999) *Restorative Justice: An Overview.* London: Home Office.

Maxwell, G.M. and Morris, A. (1993) *Families, Victims and Culture: Youth Justice in New Zealand.* Wellington: Department of Social Welfare and Institute of Criminology.

McCold, P. (2004) 'Paradigm muddle: the threat to restorative justice posed by its merger with community justice.' *Contemporary Justice Review 7*, 1, 13–35.

McKay, R. (1992) 'The resuscitation of assythment? Reparation and the Scottish Criminal Law.' *Juridical Review 3*, 242–255.

Minor, K. and Morrison, J. (1996) 'A Theoretical Study and Critique of Restorative Justice.' In B. Galaway and J. Hudson (eds) *Restorative Justice: International Perspectives*. Monsey, NY: Criminal Justice Press.

O'Connor, I. (1997) 'Models of Juvenile Justice.' In A. Borowski and I. O'Connor (eds) *Juvenile Crime, Justice and Corrections*. Melbourne: Longman.

Rowe, W. (2002) *A Meta-Analysis of Six Washington State Restorative Justice Projects: Accomplishments and Outcomes*. Washington, DC: Office of Juvenile Justice.

Schiff, M. (1998) 'The Impact of Restorative Justice Interventions on Juvenile Offenders.' In L. Walgrave and G. Bazemore (eds) *Restoring Juvenile Justice: Repairing the Harm of Youth Crime*. Monsey, NY: Criminal Justice Press.

Scottish Executive (2006) *21st Century Review of Social Work*. Edinburgh: Scottish Executive.

Sharpe, S. (1998) *Restorative Justice: A Vision for Healing and Change*. Edmonton: Edmonton Victim Offender Mediation Society.

Sherman, L., Strang, H. and Moore, D. (2000) *Recidivism Patterns in the Canberra Re-Integrative Shaming Experiments*. Canberra: Australian National University.

Umbreit, M. (1996) 'Restorative Justice through Victim–Offender Mediation: The Impact of Programs in Four Canadian Provinces.' In B. Galaway and B. Hudson (eds) *Restorative Justice: International Perspectives*. Monsey, NY: Criminal Justice Press.

Wilcox, A., Young, R. and Hoyle, C. (2004) 'An Evaluation of the Impact of Restorative Cautioning: Findings from a Reconviction Study.' *Home Office Research Findings 255*. London: Home Office.

Wright, M. (1999) *Restoring Respect for Justice*. Winchester: Waterside Press.

Wundersitz, J. (1997) 'Juvenile Justice.' In K. Hazelhurst (ed.) *Crime and Justice: An Australian Textbook in Criminology*. Sydney: Law Book Company.

Zehr, H. (2001) *Transcending: Reflections of Crime Victims*. Intercourse, PA: Good Books.

Zehr, H. (2002) *The Little Book of Restorative Justice*. Intercourse, PA: Good Books.

CHAPTER 9

Recovery in Psychosis
Moments and Levels of Collaboration
Kristjana Kristiansen

Introduction

If asked, most mental health services would today claim that a recovery orientation is central to what they provide, usually alongside stated commitments of increased user participation and person-centred planning. Closer scrutiny about what is actually happening reveals that two extremes can be identified with regard to how 'recovery' is being interpreted and acted upon. At one end, one can find services that are essentially the same as usual, but renaming current and planned efforts as 'recovery programmes'. At the other end, recovery is a protest movement of psychiatric service system survivors struggling to take back control over their lives and decisions about what kind of help is needed, and doing so outside of formalised services. Some version of any truth typically lies in the middle, and I would argue that this is true for the recovery process: services should certainly become more recovery-oriented, yet a fundamental shift in thought and action will be required in order to accomplish such intentions. Issues of expertise and control will be central in moving along this road of recovery.

A central tenet of this chapter is the belief that people with serious and often ongoing mental health distress can and do recover; they are not recovered by others. Yet traditional mental health services continue to be based on assumptions (albeit unconscious) that it is professional programmes and therapeutic interventions which are helpful when there are 'signs' of individual improvement. One key aspect in the way I have begun to understand the recovery process is that people with serious mental ill health are (or could be) essential actors in their own futures. Yet their voices often remain silenced, with their life stories seldom attended to or only understood from service perspectives and therapeutic mind-sets. Furthermore, while active agency of the affected person is a central ingredient in the recovery process, it is also all too often insufficient if actual long-term change is to occur. I have become increasingly convinced that recovery is a relational process, something that happens between the individual with mental health distress and surrounding social and societal contexts. In other words, recovery is or can be co-produced. There are many moments and levels when this can happen, or not, and this chapter presents some ideas and experiences about how this might happen more often, as well as why it should.

I will begin by describing how I understand the increasingly popular yet still elusive term 'recovery'. I then offer and discuss some implications for human service workers, and other concerned citizens, in terms of practical action. Last, some issues will be raised and explored about why doing what should be so obvious is actually quite challenging.

I will return to language-related issues, but at the start it is important to make clear what some of my ideas on 'mental health problems' are all about. Specifically, I wish to make clear that, however one understands the cause, nature and course of whatever 'craziness' is, I hope that readers will join in agreeing that individual mental distress is very real and not to be taken lightly. And, even more importantly, that the social consequences of this distress and daily struggle are often devastating, yet seldom addressed. Hence, the need for 'co-production' which has numerous opportunities to remove or lighten some of the burden from the affected individual's shoulders. When I use the phrase 'recovery in psychosis', I am referring to people with histories of psychiatric treatment and, often, long periods of hospitalisation, typically having schizophrenia-spectrum diagnoses. While I find such hegemonic psychiatric labelling an extreme challenge, I find those who consider 'madness' a mere social construction as potentially devastating for a group of fellow citizens whose very real concerns and situations might be overlooked and dismissed. I will return to this discussion later in the chapter.

Many of the following points are illustrated by comments from people I have met who have psychiatric histories and labels, and many of whom have ongoing experiences of mental health distress, yet consider themselves in recovery. I have used pseudonyms and often omit surnames, in accordance with individual wishes and corresponding ethical guidelines regarding anonymity. I often refer to these individuals as collaborative informants, and thank them very much for their vital contributions to the ways of understanding their lives, and thus helped in making this chapter possible.

Understanding 'recovery'

The term 'recovery' is often used, yet continues to be vaguely defined and interpreted in a variety of ways. Everyday usage has numerous connotations which do not help us out of this clarity-quagmire. For example, recovery can mean 'getting back to a previous position', as in recovering the economy or recovering one's balance. It can mean 'being rescued', as in ringing the recovery telephone number to get your wrecked car towed away and repaired. In health services the term is usually associated with being cured or at least showing major clinical signs of improvement. Given the lack of ongoing consensus in mental health and social services regarding this term, coupled with a near-epidemic wave of popularity especially at policy levels, I feel we should start by stating my position and describe how I understand 'being in recovery'. After all, the gap from any well-intentioned rhetoric to actual implementation is often a large and complicated leap, and it is hoped that some of the ideas may assist in narrowing this chasm.

First of all, being in recovery is about *getting on with one's life*. This is a simple and yet a fundamental starting point. This includes how one lives with the experiences of mental distress and its consequences, perhaps needing help and support now and then, but not living a life dominated by seeking or being sent on eternal quests for a cure or a better therapist. In other words, a lot of the 'condition' of mental distress may not go away, but one can still be expected and supported to participate and contribute to community life, and often quite successfully so. As one collaborative informant named David said:

> At some point, I realised I could just sort of move along, maybe at my own pace and in my own ways, but in any case get on with things…instead of hanging around the community drop-in house where I was surrounded by problems and therapy-talk.

David tells us about getting on with his life, supported, for example, by Curtis (1997) who writes: 'Recovery does not always mean that people will return to full health or retrieve all their losses, but it does mean that people can live well in spite of them.'

This is related to understanding the condition and experience of severe and often ongoing mental distress. A central element of a recovery perspective could be called *hopefulness, not chronicity*. This has been an essential step forward, given that chronicity or even progressive deterioration was long considered a definitive characteristic of the schizophrenia diagnoses. The work of (especially) psychiatrist John Strauss and colleagues challenged these Kraepelinian-based descriptions and assumptions, using data from longitudinal international studies (Strauss and Carpenter 1977), showing that the majority do improve and many considerably (see also Harding and Zahniser 1994; Harding, Zubin and Strauss 1987). Yet for a long time this research was not accepted by medical experts, who were perhaps struggling to maintain their own position and world-view (see discussions in Kristiansen 2005). Replacing a picture of chronicity with one of hopefulness is centrally related to 'getting on with life', instead of believing that life in general or one's 'condition' will never improve. As Agnes put it:

> After I got my diagnosis, I woke up every morning and felt I was in a dark hole, my body full of cement. Used all my energy to get out of bed, get through the day, and not much more. Then from somewhere, there was a light at the top of the dark pit, like a tunnel I could get through maybe.

I will return to the sources of Agnes's light later in this chapter, but at this point will mention that hopeful, upwards-oriented thinking is likely to be essential in replacing the longstanding patterns of chronicity-thinking, which have been involved in a vicious circle of self-blaming whilst also confirming the low expectations of others (Kristiansen 2005; Roets *et al.* 2007; Wolfensberger 1993).

Additionally, the notion of *citizenship not clienthood* is an essential element of thinking about people in recovery. Goffman's classical works, perhaps most notably on the nature of 'total institutions' (1961), describe how the role of 'mental patient' can be so dominant that there is little room for alternative perceptions and responses, including how one learns to consider oneself and also how one is viewed and treated by others. The importance of role perceptions and their centrality in how people are treated by their societies has been argued strongly since the recurrent writings of Wolfensberger, beginning with his seldom-read 1969 publication *The Origin and Nature of our Institutional*

Models. One is placed in the world of 'otherness', where citizenship is not an available identity or social role as long as one is seen primarily as a client in need of treatment. Have we actually progressed in the past half-century? Fredrik explained his mental ill-health experience like this: 'like a place of waiting, until you're somehow seen as ready, and then you can join everyone else'. Larry Davidson, who has a history of mental health problems himself and is now directing postgraduate and research programmes on 'recovery' at Yale University's Department of Psychiatry, uses the phrase 'a life outside of mental illness' (2003), and also reminds us that recognising fellow humanity and civil rights should be the essence of psychiatry. Being a fellow citizen living a life in recovery also means more than merely existing at the margins of society, or having unsatisfactory living conditions: citizens have entitlements such as access to decent standards of education, housing, employment, income, societal participation, and a variety of roles other than clienthood or patient.

Recovery is also about *a future, not a return.* The notion of regaining what is lost, or being 'rehabilitated' back to one's former self, is not the goal so much as finding ways of getting on with life. One man I listened to put it this way:

> I get upset looking back…so much desperation and confusion… I hurt my family so much then. I think I need to reflect more on positive things that could happen instead of what went wrong before. I'd rather stumble on ahead.

Perhaps the everyday usage of 'recovering one's balance and moving on' is useful after all? As psychiatric survivor and mental health systems consultant Patricia Deegan clearly tells us: 'For us, recovery is not about going back to who we were. It is a process of becoming new. It is a process of discovering our limits, but is also a process of discovering how those limits open upon new possibilities' (2001). And while an optimistic eye toward the future is important, and one should perhaps not strive first and foremost to regain what has been lost, part of what does happen is that one becomes more likely to be ascribed and invited into more valued social roles, expectations and responsibilities, having increased autonomy and feelings of self-worth and the like, as part of an upward spiral-effect (Curtis 1997).

Recovery involves *having more control* over one's life, including what helps or not, but also over daily life and longer-term decisions. Being in recovery includes dimensions of active agency and intention: one has to want to change and have notions of future directions, but one also typically needs support in order to proceed. Listen to Ellen's words:

> I realised it was up to me, so I learned to say no or yes and then even bigger steps, instead of being told what to do. Before, I was paralysed by insecurity and panic, but I just got analysed. Now each time I decide something, I get stronger and make bigger steps. Like, being involved in taking over management of the day-centre last year was a major sense of achievement for many of us.

Central to issues of control are issues of whose expertise is considered valid and useful, a point with far-reaching implications for co-production and change, and again, a point I will return to.

What constitutes recovery and how it happens is also *personally unique.* What is experienced as helpful or even an essential turning point may mean nothing to someone else. From listening to people's stories of recovery the seemingly tiny details of everyday life can be hugely significant, such as planting seeds in springtime or taking the neighbour's dog for a walk through autumn leaves. As James told me, 'The first time I bought a new shirt by myself after many years, I thought, wow, I can make it out here!'

Last, and quite centrally, recovery is *a process, not an outcome.* While health and social services are increasingly concerned with evaluating progress and success in terms of measuring outcomes and results, it is important to clarify that for most people with severe mental health distress this is an inappropriate way to think about their experiences or to assess service quality and relevance. Some speak about waiting for therapeutic breakthroughs that might solve their problems instead of getting on with life, as exemplified by Sonja's comment:

> I used to wait for them to change my meds, thinking this time they'll get it right…then when I moved to [another city] someone said maybe I was waiting for the wrong answers. I actually started a part-time job and wasn't very good at it, but it was good medicine.

Recovery is not a clinical goal or therapeutic outcome, but rather an ongoing, dynamic process. Therefore, I use the phrase 'in recovery in psychosis', not necessarily having recovered from it. A life in recovery is a journey, often along *a bumpy road,* and, as with life, for most people a recovery process will have its ups and downs. Lillian talked about how she wished she knew that most people had 'down' times and 'bad' days, that such experiences were 'normal' and not part of her 'mental health syndrome'. She described learning that other people also had very stressful and painful times as one of her 'most therapeutic moments'.

In a book such as this about 'welfare', it may be interesting to note that the English root of this word is from the Nordic 'velferd', which means to travel well and safely, as in the now out-of-date British goodbye greeting 'fare-thee-well', or as the 'goodbye' greeting in Norway: 'Far vel!' Some roads are well taken alone, even some of the bumpy parts. Yet the recovery road is not meant to be taken alone for most people, although some of its steps may be, because *the recovery process is social*. It is not something that happens inside the individual's mind or body, and not something that can be fixed or cured solely through individually located interventions. Recovery is best seen as a social journey, in interaction with other nearby people and the whole of society, and therefore a journey with many unused opportunities for collaboration: moments and levels for co-production.

Moving towards practical action

This section offers some ideas that may be helpful for human service workers in moving towards 'co-producing' recovery, building on what has been presented thus far and also on some of my other experiences in getting to know and live with people who have had some very rough times living with severe and often ongoing mental distress.

First, I believe that, if any significant change is to occur, there must be a fundamental change in the *mind-sets* of human service workers and their societies. Who 'are' people with long histories of serious mental distress? What are their most important needs? What is the role of services (or not) in moving forward? Underlying any attempt to address such huge questions will be a foundation of *humility*, which I feel is a necessary but probably insufficient element of this much-needed mind-set change.

The nature and origin of serious mental distress is still largely dominated by a medical culture, a tradition searching for causality, valid and reliable diagnoses, subsequent treatments, and relief if not cure. This kind of thinking has shaped and continues to maintain the beliefs of the general public, taught in a number of direct and indirect ways to trust its sanctioned experts and accept their accompanying mind-sets, albeit unknowingly. Present-day mental health services herald client-centredness and interdisciplinary team-work, with psychiatric hegemonic ghosts lingering on in the nearby shadows. The recovery process, in any case, is not a view centred on client/patient roles, diagnostic processes, therapeutic relationships etc., but rather revolves around genuinely being able to see and believe in the person who is experiencing distress (see especially the work by Larry Davidson and Patricia Deegan), while also addressing their societal situations. On the one hand, one can find service workers who believe that a clinical focus is primarily what is needed, as well as being one's proper job purview. There seems to be an assumption, occasionally even explicitly stated, that conditions such as social isolation and poverty will somehow be resolved or at least significantly alleviated once the 'illness' is cured. Alternatively, or at least apparently so, there are those who profess and believe that they are actually seeing and dealing with the person and his/her situation in more holistic ways. Yet these approaches typically continue to locate the problem and potential solutions within the individual person since, even when broader situations are considered, it is the individual's own environments that are taken into account.

Expanding and addressing the origin and nature of 'the problem' is the first part of mind-set change: recovery is about getting on with life, not about getting cured or rehabilitated so that one can...perhaps...someday...get on with life. It is also to a great extent about ownership of problem-definition and resultant thinking about priorities. In describing the differences between various mind-sets, Phil summed up two varying starting points this way when describing his meetings with psychiatrists: 'Before, I was discounted as one with delusions of grandeur...now we are a team, working together on a project called Phil.'

Why mention humility in a discussion about mind-sets? In a book about co-production, and more specifically here about the recovery process? I do so because I believe that it is often when someone describes things that seem impossible that that 'someone' may be most in need of being very humbly and seriously listened to: that a central need for that person may be about being believed when describing feelings and situations and experiences that seem to others so unbelievable. Margret, for example, mentioned that her support worker had often acknowledged that Margret's anxiety was clearly very debilitating in her daily life, and that her economic worries were certainly justifiable, but Margret wondered if this support worker really had any chance of truly understanding:

> She's never been so scared and overwhelmed by panic that she can't leave her house for weeks, like with me...and she knows I can't pay my bills, but does she have any idea what being poor all the time feels like?

And, as Henrik said:

> I can't stand social workers who learned somewhere to nod their head at some empathetic angle and say they understand…they can't possibly understand what my life has been like… One of the first guys who really helped me said he couldn't imagine what I was going through… He was apologising, like he was supposed to know… I thought, 'At last, someone who's honest!'

The sort of humility needed by Margret or Henrik is much deeper than empathy or 'reflexive therapeutic thinking'. Henrik later added:

> He didn't think 'Yikes, thank god that's not me', I mean he wasn't afraid of me…and he didn't feel sorry or sad…he just listened and he heard me. I shouldn't say 'just' listened, but I mean so many others never have… He really saw the person inside me that is me!

The second point of discussion in this section gets its sub-title from one of our collaborating informants, who declared at a regional meeting of service-users and survivors: *'Partnership yes please, empowerment no thanks!'* People have been successfully getting on with their often very distressing mental health problems for ages, and while they these days describe themselves as being in recovery, they rarely mention services or providers as helpful or significant (Glover 2005). Yet there are some exceptions, or critical moments, that can occur in a helping relationship (see, for example, discussions in Borg and Kristiansen 2004; Trivedi and Wykes 2002). As Trish Burnett from the Scottish Recovery Movement (www.scottishrecovery.net) stated: 'For me, recovery is like climbing a mountain…you need a map and the right equipment as well as someone to guide you.' In the end, Trish has to climb her mountain, but equipment and a map and a guide could be helpful and even necessary. The mountain-metaphor may be overwhelming for many who experience recovery as an up-and-down, bumpy road. But could we all agree that the journey to recovery would not be helped if the only equipment offered up the mountain or along the unknown road to the future was a new wonder-drug or a place at the day-centre, the only map was your personal social network drawn on paper by your assigned social worker, and the guide was a nurse with extra qualifications in community mental health but afraid of heights and forests?

Power is a central ingredient of a recovery-orientation. The much acclaimed hope of human service workers to 'empower' others quite clearly implies who has the power to start with. But recovery is about attaining or regaining control over one's life and one's distress, and not being given it by others. The possibilities and moments for partnership around power-shifting are both numerous and fragile, requiring a give–take balance where the vulnerable person is, it is hoped, the more active and initiating one. The service worker's role should be to learn to recognise and support opportunities for inviting and engaging, rather than giving or assigning power and control. Janet said, 'At first, I thought, well, they're giving me enough rope to hang myself…then I realised they were opening doors and windows, but only if I took the chance, that it was up to me and that I could do it.'

One of the largest potential sources of power that service workers have is related to hope. Succinctly and profoundly, Helen Glover has called human service workers 'holders of hope' (2002), and I support her contention that offering hope should be central to anyone attempting a 'recovery partnership'. Providing and instilling hope in others who have experienced a lifetime of hopelessness may be essential to even start the recovery process. The hope-ingredient of the recovery process may be particularly important for people who have long been clinically described and treated as hopeless, such as those with labels of schizophrenia, where chronicity has long been a defining characteristic of the diagnosis. Research (Kristiansen 2005) has identified four aspects of hope that are important experiences for individuals: *believing me* (trusting that my experiences are real, even when I may not be sure myself); *believing in me* (that I can change); *believing that my future can be different* (that my life in general can improve); and *believing that I can make a difference in my future* (that some of what needs to change can be done by me, no matter how bad things seem today). Often, 'believing me' and 'believing in me' are necessary prerequisites for moving into actual and future changes. How to transmit such messages to those who seek or may need them is, however, no easy task, and not one lightly built into training courses for well-intentioned service providers. In fact, Henrik's previously mentioned comment about empathic head-nodding exemplifies how sad the experienced consequences might be, as if learning head-nodding is the way to provide a message of understanding and empathy.

Partnership is also about learning together. Helen Glover described a health care worker who said that most clients are happy to be told what to do and may even want no responsibility for answers, and found it quite refreshing that Helen herself wanted to be very active in own-care decisions (2005). She continues that this service provider felt they had a partnership where they each learned from each other. Thus, in addition to co-producing recovery, one is also co-producing knowledge and mutual learning.

Additionally, there are *many levels* for collaboration and co-production in recovery processes. Part of this may be in partnership, but much may also involve service workers and other citizens advocating for societal changes and addressing conditions that are extremely distressful and potentially devastating for people with mental health histories and labels, yet which are not clinical or therapeutic issues. For example, being in recovery includes being perceived and treated as a citizen with social roles and civil rights, and accomplishing this will involve other people who typically already have valued social roles and are able to use their citizenship rights for change. Being in recovery also means being included in society, not just hanging around on the fringes struggling to survive. It includes having a decent standard of living conditions (education, income, housing, employment), which will usually also require action from others. Recovery is also a social process, such that other people, and often not paid human service workers, may need to invite and support people living at society's margins to join in and participate. Again, there are many moments and levels for this to occur and Inge's comment is a good illustration:

> For years we weren't allowed to attend that [local event]…not really a legal thing, just that they didn't want us from the [psychiatric] hospital there. One year Jon-Petter and his wife invited me and a friend of mine, and it was fun and we didn't eat anybody [laughs]…after that more and more people started to attend. People found out we were really okay, and we found out life out there wasn't so scary!

Some additional challenges

This section offers some reflections on why doing what should be so obvious seems to be so difficult.

First of all there is the confusion and lack of consensus about what recovery actually is, and who should decide. Is *roominess in discourse* good news or bad news? Lack of clarity and subsequent lack of utility in terms of immediate applicability may be disturbing to many. Not surprisingly, many human service workers want to know how to use new ideas in their daily work with people, and are typically not paid for time spent reflecting or even thinking at critical levels deep enough to rock the boat. Yet some knowledge takes time to develop and may not have immediate application, leaving concepts and ideas unclear but also open for further scrutiny. Concept roominess also provides space for debates which may be sorely needed. Such debates often invite and create polarisations which have important functions in early phases of concept clarification and refinement, especially in terms of differences that can be sorted out or not. But such polarisations can also lead to schisms and chasms which are difficult to mend and build bridges across. As disabled activist and scholar Tom Shakespeare has repeatedly pointed out, early 'social model' writings quite profoundly and justifiably challenged medical hegemony regarding understanding what 'disability' was all about, yet often went so far as to downplay or even deny the painful daily realities of actual impairments (2004, 2006). Aside from a contentious issue in the UK disability studies arena, the impairment–disability debate is mainly an ontological question of how one understands the 'real' world. This is especially so at the crossroads where disability politics meets science and philosophy (Vehmas 2008).

The ways of understanding the recovery process and the nature of 'madness' are current examples of such polarisations and debates, including defining who has what problem and what 'it' should be named. Psychiatric labelling and the life-dominating mental patient role have long led to many negative consequences, such as social stigma or inequality in employment. Some propose label-removal as the solution, partly based on the belief that mental illness is merely a social construction. But not having one's individual distress recognised and somehow named could lead to serious difficulties (Kristiansen 2005; Söder 2004), including having one's needs for individual supports or benefits overlooked or denied. Surely addressing loneliness and poverty, which are two common experiences for people with long-term mental health distress, cannot be solved by mere category-deconstruction and label-removal? Narrowing understandings of disability or mental disorder to purely social issues is likely to be as limiting as only viewing such as bio-medical conditions or psycho-emotional states. I support those who view the experience and situation as multi-dimensional, such as Shakespeare (2006) and Davidson and Strauss (1995), who argue for more complex frames when thinking about disability, disorder, health and recovery.

Regardless of one's aetiological perspective concerning the nature and origin of 'madness', that something is very 'real' for the affected individual (I could call it the impairment) and not to be taken lightly. I also have come to believe that, while this personal distress may at times be devastating, the social consequences and associated situations are typically even more disabling and accumulative. And because we see the recovery process (or lack of) as a social process, there are again many levels and moments for collaborative thinking and action.

And now some ideas on knowledge and expertise. On the one hand, I believe that subjective, lived experience is an important knowledge source (Davidson 2003; Deegan 1988; Kristiansen 2005; Strauss 1996; Trivedi and Wykes 2002). Again, this may be especially important for many people with histories of schizophrenia-labels, since their subjective voices have long been described as fragmented, untrustworthy and out of touch with reality. To the extent they have been listened to, it has been primarily to search for signs and symptoms to match them with diagnostic categories as a step toward treatment (which was often about symptom alleviation, since chronicity and even progressive deterioration were syndrome-descriptors).

Of course I believe that long-silenced voices should be seriously listened to, and from non-clinical perspectives. However, on another extreme, one can find service user groups and politically correct service providers who think solutions should only be those articulated by the wishes and demands of the person in need. An interesting situation!? How does anyone actually know if what one wants and asks for is actually what one 'needs'? And who should decide? What is important to find out, how can we find out, and who needs to know what and for what purpose? Does theory have a place in social change, and if so, where does theory come from and how?

These are of course fundamental questions of ontology and epistemology, and space here does not allow much delving deeper into this important subject matter. Yet I will state one thing that is both somewhat concrete and somewhat controversial: I believe that the subjective experience and voice of those with lived experience is a very valuable and often under-utilised source of knowledge, yet that this is likely to be insufficient for societal change. Instead I would argue that subjective experiences and assessments of what is going on should be coupled with objective information, for example concrete data about living conditions. The rationale for this is not to confirm or refute the subjective experiences, but to supplement the picture of what is real. My experience is that often those who have lived lives with very little access to decent living conditions, for example, may be content to get just a little bit more, rather than what they may deserve as fellow citizens. In other words, the most disadvantaged in society may wish and demand much less than what average citizens would consider a basic human need or civil right.

An everyday life perspective is essential

I have come to believe that what I would call an everyday life perspective appears to be an essential dimension of the needed mind-set changes referred to earlier. Part of this is connected to what is also known as a living conditions approach: that is, looking at how and where people live their daily lives. Whatever is happening (or not) with people with mental health problems, it occurs in these everyday life, social contexts. This of course includes people who are alone and lonely, since the exclusion process is also a social one. It is therefore within social contexts and everyday life that I believe people and their situations need to be understood and supported.

An everyday life orientation is helpful in shifting one's gaze, our ways of thinking and responding. First of all, a person-not-patient view is more likely: our gaze shifts from the pathological and problematic to daily life activities and conditions in society. Second, a whole life picture gives a larger context for analysis, interpretation and solution-finding than does an individual-based assessment. Resources and opportunities to build on are likely to be at the meeting points between the individual and the society. An everyday life orientation is also connected to civil rights, acknowledging people's personhood and citizenship (not just 'user/consumer involvement'). In Norway living conditions surveys are specifically used to unveil patterns of inequality for certain vulnerable groups of citizens, and are directly linked to social policy change in areas such as housing, education and employment (Tøssebro and Kittelsaa 2004).

One of the challenges of this perspective for service providers is the issue of purview: if everyday life is an essential perspective, whose domain is it? After all, we do not want to train a generation of 'private-space invaders', assessing all life domains in hopes of uncovering possibilities for recovery potential. The answer to such a question may have little difference for the individual who needs practical help or even a bit of ongoing advice and support. But a danger may be that professionals are likely to engage in territorial disputes, ranging from 'We've been visiting people in their homes for decades' to 'We know he's poor and lonely, but I work for the supported employment office so it's not my re-sponsibility'. This entire area presents numerous challenges, none of which is easily resolved. Let us rather think of the many possibilities and often apparently small moments for collaboration. Everyday life is elusive and deceptive: it is both simple and yet complex.

The paradox of triviality

A major challenge in thinking about the recovery process in the midst of everyday life is that trivial things and events are not so trivial after all. Small things do count, and may be significant turning points in an individual's journey in recovery. They may be happenings so tiny as to remain unseen by the outsider. The apparently mundane is after all quite complex, especially in social contexts. So much of everyday life is taken for granted that it risks being unnamed and invisible. Thus, many moments for discovery of such as co-production pass all of us by. 'Common sense is unfortunately not so common, and the obvious is not always so obvious', as one of our collaborating informants, Julie, so brilliantly phrased it.

Recovery is unique and personal, and so will be the small bits of the process, varying from individual to individual. This means that service delivery cannot design systemic solutions or models, which would require norms and standards, and have little room for surprises and creative use of opportunity. This is a central paradox of putting a recovery orientation into practice.

Some concluding comments and reflections

Recovery is in danger of becoming a fragmented effort that may slip into dilution. Increasingly one finds on the one hand the radical disability/survivor spokespeople arguing and demanding more control and often total liberation from formalised services. This is perhaps not surprising when they often continue to experience being the weaker, dependent, 'needy' party when attempting partnership. In an era where most services eagerly nod that 'recovery' is something they do or have been doing all along, one can see the many rhetorical twists that seem to indicate co-opting yet another grass-roots movement. Services re-label themselves as recovery-orientated, yet still focus on symptom management, monitoring and relapse-prevention. Helen Glover clearly tells us to return to essential principles, not just embrace the term, and partnership is one of these essentials (2005). Whose side needs to change, and where are the moments and levels for collaborative efforts?

Critical moments for change may be difficult to discover because they appear so small or so outside what is generally considered a service purview ('You bought a pet canary-bird, and it changed your life?'). Other moments seem so overwhelmingly huge or impossible to confront, or again 'not really my job', such as changing psychiatric mind-sets or altering societal attitudes. However, I believe that everyday life for each one of us is full of moments that are both small and large, and that each one of us has choices about making life different for ourselves as well as for others: in other words, co-producing better societies?

Acknowledgements

This chapter should have been more carefully referenced – after a while, one's thinking becomes quite intertwined with one's colleagues and mentors. I in any case owe much to the work and writings of John Strauss, Larry Davidson, Courtney Harding (USA), Marit Borg (Norway), Helen Glover (Australia), and for many years the writings of Wolf Wolfensberger (Germany and USA) and probably many others. Thank you. And especially thank you to the people with mental health problems who shared their lives and experiences, often in the midst of very distressing times for them: without each of you, the knowledge presented in this chapter would be incomplete, and certainly not co-produced.

References

Borg, M. and Kristiansen, K. (2004) 'Recovery-oriented professionals: helping relationships in mental health services.' *Journal of Mental Health 13*, 5, 495–505.

Curtis, L. (1997) *New Directions: International Overview of Best Practices in Recovery and Rehabilitation Services for People with Serious Mental Illness, A Discussion Paper.* New Zealand: The Commission to Inform the Development of a National Blueprint for Mental Health Services.

Davidson, L. (2003) *Living Outside of Mental Illness: Qualitative Studies of Recovery in Schizophrenia.* New York, NY: New York University Press.

Davidson, L. and Strauss, J. (1995) 'Beyond the biopsychosocial model: integrating disorder, health, and recovery.' *Psychiatry 85*, 44–54.

Deegan, P. (1988) 'Recovery: the lived experience of rehabilitation.' *Psychosocial Rehabilitation Journal 11*, 4, 11–19.

Deegan, P. (2001) *Recovery as a Self-Directed Process of Healing and Transformation.* Massachusetts, NE: Pat Deegan and Associates.

Glover, H. (2002) *Developing a Recovery Platform for Mental Health Service Delivery for People with Mental Illness/Distress in England.* Working paper. London: National Institute of Mental Health.

Glover, H. (2005) 'Recovery-based service delivery: are we ready to transform the words into a paradigm shift?' *Australian E-Journal for the Advancement of Mental Health 4*, 3, 1–4.

Goffman, E. (1961) *Asylums*. Englewood Cliffs, NJ: Penguin Books.

Harding, C. and Zahniser, J. (1994) 'Empirical correction of seven myths about schizophrenia with implications for treatment.' *Acta Psychiatrica Scandinavica 90*, suppl. 384, 140–146.

Harding, C., Zubin, J. and Strauss, J. (1987) 'Chronicity in schizophrenia: fact, partial fact, or artifact?' *Hospital and Community Psychiatry 38*, 5, 477–486.

Kristiansen, K. (2005) 'Owners of Chemistry, Hope and Evidence.' In A. Gustavsson, J. Sandvin, R. Traustadóttir and J. Tøssebro (eds) *Resistance, Reflection, and Change: Disability Research in the Nordic Countries*. Lund: Lund University Press.

Roets, G., Kristiansen, K., VanHove, G. and Vandersplassen, W. (2007) 'Living through exposure to toxic psychiatric orthodoxies: exploring narratives of people with mental health problems who are looking for employment.' *Disability and Society 22*, 83, 267–281.

Shakespeare, T. (2004) 'Social models of disability and other life strategies.' *Scandinavian Journal of Disability Research 6*, 1, 8–21.

Shakespeare, T. (2006) *Disability Rights and Wrongs*. London: Routledge.

Söder, M. (2004) 'Why Head-Counting?' In J. Tøssebro and A. Kittelsaa (eds) *Exploring the Living Conditions of Disabled People*. Lund: Lund University Press.

Strauss, J. (1996) 'Subjectivity.' *Journal of Nervous and Mental Disease 184*, 4, 205–212.

Strauss, J. and Carpenter, W.T. (1977) 'Prediction of outcome in schizophrenia.' *Archives of General Psychiatry 34*, 159–163.

Tøssebro, J. and Kittelsaa, A. (eds) (2004) *Exploring the Living Conditions of Disabled People*. Lund: Lund University Press.

Trivedi, P. and Wykes, T. (2002) 'From passive subjects to equal partners: user involvement in research – a review.' *British Journal of Psychiatry 181*, 468–472.

Vehmas, S. (2008) 'Philosophy and science: the axes of evil in disability studies?' *Journal of Medical Ethics*, forthcoming.

Wolfensberger, W. (1969) *The Origin and Nature of our Institutional Models*. Syracuse, NY: Human Policy Press.

Wolfensberger, W. (1993) *Social Role Valorization*. Syracuse, NY: Syracuse University Press.

Endnote

This is what strikes us as editors of this volume in reflecting on the preceding contributions.

Each chapter describes a context for co-production – whether a specific local or national project, a particular method or professional discipline, a formal service delivery structure or an explicit philosophical approach.

Each context is different, but they share some family resemblances; for example:

- A healthy respect for people's capacity to define what is important, to make changes, to be part of the solution; this is not anti-professional but a different world-view that takes account of capacities and strengths of individuals and communities.

- A focus on authentic relationship between help-giver and help-taker; engagement rather than 'objectivity' at the core.

- Being grounded in, and working with, the wider community – rather than drawing the individual into a separate 'service land'; co-production complements rather than replaces specialist services which can then target their resources differently.

- An uneasy relationship with 'the mainstream' – dancing the thin line between incorporation and marginalisation, becoming diluted and being too hard to swallow.

- An emphasis on facilitating a process, with perceptions and possibilities changing over time, rather than simply delivering a product; having the discretion to respond to creative moments; having a light bureaucratic touch.

- Success requires unusual skill, commitment and attention to detail; a willingness to share power by 'letting go' of the need to be right, but retaining the authority to advise and guide, and the willingness to go back in if necessary without saying 'I told you so'.

Given this, it's not hard to see why extending and embedding co-production within the service system presents a conceptual and practical challenge.

The *Report of the 21st Century Review of Social Work* (Scottish Executive 2006) could be seen as an attempt to take up this challenge. If the personalisation and participation agenda is to be taken forward, and if propositions about partnership and citizenship are to be taken seriously, it will be necessary to:

- reinstate relationship working at the heart of the health and social care agenda

- understand that the co-production agenda, with its small-scale beginnings, is one of transformational change despite its natural locus amongst front-line resources

- install the hardware as well as the software to support co-production so that co-production 'counterfeits' do not take root in the risk-averse, regulatory culture of our services

- be alert to the risks of exploitation, shifting the burden of care and responsibility on to families and of 'covert operations' by which co-production is used as a justification for the status quo

- develop a sophisticated approach to balancing the need for safeguarding vulnerable people within a philosophy of self-direction and self-management

- resist the temptation to create yet another category of potential professionals – SVQs for mentors, for local area coordinators, for recovery buddies – that distracts from the central focus of relationships, power and proximity that characterise co-production

- recognise that individualised funding, without input from people who are 'expert' in their own problems, will not achieve individualised services

- invest in leadership but at all levels individual, professional and strategic, building capacity to develop and challenge a twenty-first-century reconfiguration of service, citizenship and responsibility.

The ways of working described in this book can co-exist alongside traditional ways of working. A modest amount of innovation can occur without displacing existing practices or tipping the system. Indeed well-established methods can be resilient in the face of new evidence and aspiration, colonising and reinventing new ideas in their own image. Anyone embarking on co-production should be prepared to dig in for the long haul.

Alongside the alert to the 'colonising' capacity of service systems sits the alert to opportunism within the political system, or whatever party complexion, that sees in co-production the prospect of shifting the 'burden of welfare' on to the shoulders of its recipients. Co-production is about forging new forms of working relationships, not abrogating responsibility.

Co-production isn't a magical solution to the seemingly intractable problem of why services set out with good intentions but end up too often with poor results. It does, however, invite professionals to reconsider the 'We'll fix it' response to people requiring services and to become intolerant of systemic incompetence. A shared recognition of the limitations of the human service system is the first step in co-creating more sustaining and sustainable communities.

Co-production is not a model: it is a philosophy. As the contributions in this collection demonstrate, it is a positive affirmation that people can develop their own futures with the support of others including professionals.

Reference

Scottish Executive (2006) *Changing Lives: Report of the 21st Century Social Work Review.* Edinburgh: Scottish Executive.

The Contributors

Eddie Bartnik has a very broad and long-term perspective on supporting people with disabilities and their families, having worked in the field for 30 years holding a range of senior government positions in policy, funding and service delivery. He was the inaugural Director of Disability Program Policy and Funding at the time of the formation of the Disability Services Commission in Western Australia. He worked to establish a coherent policy and funding framework for the non government sector the first of its kind in Australia that covered all areas of disability. Eddie has had a major leadership role with the state-wide Local Area Coordination (LAC) programme, which now supports more than 8000 people with disabilities and their families throughout Western Australia, and also operates in a number of other states and countries. He has also been a leader in the reform of services in Western Australia, focusing on individualised and direct funding mechanisms to increase choice and control, as well as initiatives to strengthen individual and family leadership and community engagement. In addition to overseeing the completion of the LAC network across Western Australia, Eddie in recent years has presented conference papers and consulted with families, community groups and governments across Australia, as well as in the UK, Holland, Poland, the USA, Canada and New Zealand.

Ron Chalmers is the Acting Director General of the WA Disability Services Commission following nine years as the Country Services Director with the Commission. He has a background in teaching and educational administration and became involved in disability services in 1991 as a Local Area Coordinator Supervisor for the Upper Great Southern area of Western Australia. Dr Chalmers has extensive experience in the development and expansion of the Commission's Local Area Coordination programme and in the needs of people living in rural communities. His experience in disability services spans the full range of roles from field-based work through to running the Western Australian Disability Services Commission (2006–7). He holds a Masters degree in educational leadership and a PhD enquiring into the inclusion of children with severe and profound disabilities into mainstream schooling.

Steve Coulson has worked for 20 years with people with learning difficulties and their families. At Edinburgh Development Group his work has focused on young people planning for good lives after school. He is the co-author of *The Big Plan – A Good Life after School.*

James Cox is employed by the City of Edinburgh Council Children and Families Department as a Family Group Conference Coordinator. He is also seconded part time as a Professional Adviser to the Scottish Executive (Directorate for Children, Young People and Social Care).

Susan Hunter lectures in social work at the University of Edinburgh. She has teaching responsibilities and research interests in the areas of learning disabilities and ageing. She is also active in a number of voluntary organisations including Scottish Human Services, whose work is particularly reflected in this volume.

Kristjana Kristiansen is an Associate Professor, Department of Social Work and Health Sciences, Norwegian University of Science and Technology, in Trondheim, Norway, where she teaches research methods, disability studies and community mental health work at the post-graduate level. She originally trained as a psychologist, and completed her doctoral studies in public health. Her current research interests are everyday life studies for people with serious mental distress and participatory research methodologies, and has published and lectured widely on these topics.

James Mulholland, after having had a triple heart by-pass operation in 1996, was looking for some ongoing support with his rehabilitation and found 'Braveheart'. This has become a fantastic source of support, having been involved as a supportee, a mentor and now currently Chair of the organisation. Prior to joining Braveheart, he had retired in 1994 after 30 years' service in the aero engineering industry with Rolls Royce plc.

Jane Pagler, after working 30 years in various practitioner and management roles in social care settings, established her own business in 2003 as an independent business adviser. She has a variety of paid and voluntary roles ranging from direct client work to strategic support for not-for-profit organisations. She particularly enjoys supporting people with impairments to set up their own businesses. Jane has a hearing impairment and lives in Cardiff with her partner.

Carl Poll started KeyRing Living Support Networks in 1990. Since leaving KeyRing he has worked with in Control, the national programme that is developing a new model of social care – Self-Directed Support. He is in Control's Director of Communications. Over recent years he has contributed to raising a national debate on the meaning of citizenship for marginalised people, organising seminal conferences with speakers such as John McKnight from Chicago and Varun Vidyarthi from Lucknow, India.

Pete Ritchie trained as a social worker and community worker. The focus of his work has been promoting inclusion and social justice for people at risk of exclusion, in particular people with a learning disability.

Bill Whyte is Professor of Social Work Studies in Criminal and Youth Justice at the University of Edinburgh and Director of the Criminal Justice Social Work Development Centre for Scotland, Universities of Edinburgh and Stirling. He has worked as a social work manager and field social worker in the Lothians area, as a residential care worker in a (former List D) residential school, as an independent chair of child protection for a small local authority and currently provides advice and consultancy to managers and workers in criminal justice social work, youth social work and to other related professionals.

Subject Index

Author Index